Let us hope that before the last sands have run out from beneath the feet of the years of the nineteenth century it will have become a model of its kind, and that upon the centennial of its anniversary it will be a hospital which shall still compare favorably, not only in structure and arrangement, but also in results achieved, with any other institution of like character in existence.

John Shaw Billings,
address at the opening of
The Johns Hopkins Hospital,
May 1889

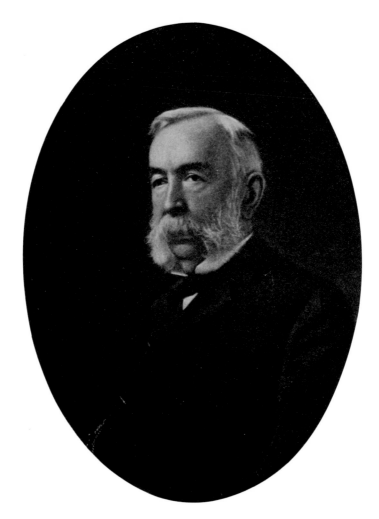

Daniel C. Gilman

A Model of Its Kind

Volume II
A PICTORIAL HISTORY OF MEDICINE
AT JOHNS HOPKINS

*A. McGehee Harvey, Gert H. Brieger, Susan L. Abrams,
Jonathan M. Fishbein, and Victor A. McKusick*

The Johns Hopkins University Press
Baltimore and London

©1989 The Johns Hopkins University Press
All rights reserved
Printed in the United States of America
The Johns Hopkins University Press
701 West 40th Street
Baltimore, MD 21211
The Johns Hopkins Press Ltd., London

The paper used in this publication meets the minimum requirements of
American National Standard for Information Sciences—Permanence of
Paper for Printed Library Materials, ANSI Z39.48-1984.

Library of Congress Cataloging-in-Publication Data

A Model of its kind.

Includes index.
Contents: v. 1. A centennial history of medicine at Johns Hopkins—
v. 2. A pictorial history of medicine at Johns Hopkins.
1. Johns Hopkins Medical School–History. I. Harvey,
A. McGehee (Abner McGehee), 1911–
R747.J62M63   1989   610'.7'117526   88-46064
ISBN 0-8018-3794-4 (v. 1 : alk. paper)
ISBN 0-8018-3816-9 (v. 2 : alk paper)

CONTENTS

ACKNOWLEDGMENTS

Our deep appreciation goes to the staff of the Alan Mason Chesney Medical Archives, especially Gerard Shorb, whose detailed knowledge of the Archives' photograph collection and whose persistence in finding dozens of elusive images made this book possible.

We wish to thank Betty Liggett Cuthbert, R.N., and the Johns Hopkins Nurses' Alumnae Association, Inc., for their willingness to share information and illustrations from their slide-tape presentation on the history of the School of Nursing. We also thank W. W. Scott, M.D., for the photograph of Dr. Young, and Linda Mishkin of the Office of Public Affairs for her help in locating and attributing photographs.

Our thanks also to Daniel M. Fox for letting us read the galleys of his book, *Photographing Medicine* (Westport, Conn.: Greenwood Press, 1988).

Above all, our thanks to Thomas Stiltz, who designed both this book and its companion volume.

A Model of Its Kind

Volume II
A PICTORIAL HISTORY OF MEDICINE
AT JOHNS HOPKINS

INTRODUCTION

"If I could tell the story in words, I wouldn't need to lug a camera," the American photographer Lewis Hine once wrote.[1] And James Agee, in his book *Let Us Now Praise Famous Men*, expressed a similar view when he said, "If I could do it, I'd do no writing at all here. It would be photographs."[2] Photographs convey a different kind of information from mere words—sharply different details about the evolution of medical practice, teaching, and the quest for knowledge. Because photographs help to tell the story more fully, they make the history of Hopkins more vivid, more concrete, more dramatic.

At the center of this history are the master teachers, investigators, and clinicians who have populated Hopkins since its inception. It was the presence of these individuals that led Alan Gregg to refer to Hopkins' "heritage of excellence," a quality that emerges from "the close but entirely free association of really superior people."[3] As the word *heritage* implies, the students trained by these masters have gone on to become masters themselves.

Indeed, the original residency system at Hopkins was predicated on the idea that one person would become "the resident," remaining at Hopkins for long enough to become not simply a fully trained practitioner but also a superior physician and teacher. The classic example was William S. Thayer, who lived in the hospital as Osler's second-in-command for seven years. In the 1930s, Deryl Hart became professor of surgery at Duke University immediately after completing his surgical residency at Hopkins.

The Alan Mason Chesney Medical Archives of the Johns Hopkins Medical Institutions, the source of most of the pictures in this volume, is rich in photographs of these masters. This volume contains many of these photographs, which show William Osler, William S. Halsted, Howard A. Kelly and their successors in characteristic poses, instructing small and large groups of students, at the bedside, in the lecture-hall, and in the laboratory. Here is the essence of medicine at Hopkins: the faculty members, house officers, and students all engaging in "learning by doing."

In choosing the photographs for this volume, an objective has been to show the changes in the working spaces of the hospital and medical school. The plot of land that houses the hospital and medical school has been filled in a variety of ways throughout the past century, and these pictures are intended to document not only the sequential structural changes but changes in the way medicine has been practiced and investigated here as well.

Most of these photographs were selected from the more than ten thousand prints in the archives. Many have been printed previously, but in this companion to the first volume, they are printed together in one place for the first time.

Like most institutional collections, the holdings of the archives are rich in some kinds of pictures, poor in others. There is, for instance, an overabundance of posed group photographs. These include class pictures, faculty and staff photos, laboratory groups, nursing teams, and the like. There are also hundreds of individual portraits, hundreds of views of buildings being constructed or torn down, of clinics, laboratories, hospital rooms, and dormitory rooms.

The collection nevertheless has gaps. Although women were an important part of the medical school from its inception, the collection gives inadequate evidence of their important role. There are many excellent photographs of nursing activities, and all the class pictures include the women students, but in the truly revealing photographs—the ones that depict action in medicine, whether practice, learning, or research—there are few that include, much less feature, women.

Overall, the photographs for this volume have been chosen to display the many facets of medicine at Johns Hopkins over the past century by showing the spaces in which they took place. The intention has been to focus especially on the working spaces—those used for teaching, for learning, for caring, for curing, and for the pursuit of new knowledge to advance the scientific basis of medical practice.

The camera serves much more fully than words to record architectural style and the arrangement of internal space and to display the use of buildings. Thus one is able to *see* learning or treatment in progress, not merely to read a verbal description. The photographs in this volume offer, in the words of John Collier, Jr., and Malcolm Collier, a "cultural inventory" of medicine at Hopkins. The Colliers applied this concept to the home. "The photographic inventory," they wrote, "can record not only the range of artifacts in a home but also their relationship to each other, the style of their placement in space, all the aspects that define and express the way in which people use and order their space and possessions."[4]

The concept of a "cultural inventory" can also be applied to an institution. In these photographs, the "artifacts" are the medical equipment, the arrangement of furniture, and the features of the buildings themselves. Thus the photographs depict the ways in which the faculty, staff, and patients inhabit the space and use these artifacts. What are the physicians wearing? How are they grouped around the patient? What are the spatial relationships among nurses, physicians, and patients? How have these changed over the years, and what does such information convey? In the laboratory, what equipment appears? Where are the assistants, and what are they shown to be doing? In sum, what was it like to be a patient, a nurse, a doctor, a student, a staff member at Hopkins?

For many historical periods, photographs have added an important, if not a crucial, dimension to historical understanding. Individual memories of the Great Depression have been supplemented by the moving portraits of families on the road or of farms being swallowed up by sandstorms. The pictures of the Farm Security Administration, taken by photographers such as Dorothea Lange, Arthur Rothstein, Walker Evans, and Russell Lee, have come to represent the period, not only in the vision of it but in the understanding of it as well.[5]

Although photographs are historical documents in themselves, they require verbal clues for their interpretation. Neither words nor pictures can stand alone. In the Hopkins collection, many pictures are without caption, and what captions were available were often limited to a very few words of identification. Some captions have been amplified with the words of contemporaries of the pictorial scenes; in other cases, readers will recognize those portrayed and will be able to supply captions for themselves.

The final determinant of meaning in a photograph is thus the perception of the viewer himself. No matter how detailed are the descriptions of the photographs in the following pages, each viewer will bring an additional, personal point of view to what is shown or said.

The halftone print was introduced in about 1890, a development that produced what the historian Neil Harris has called an "iconographical revolution." This milestone in the art and science of photography coincided with the founding and early years of the Johns Hopkins Hospital and School of Medicine. In a real sense, therefore, photography and Hopkins grew up together. "The single generation of Americans living between 1885 and 1910 went through an experience of visual reorientation that had few earlier precedents," Harris wrote.[6]

The growth of Hopkins was thus depicted in a growing number of photographs. The increasing affluence of the middle class in American society encouraged the growth in popularity of informal photographs. Cameras became simpler and faster to operate, and now anyone could be "a photographer."[7] The frozen, richly detailed photographs of the new hospital taken by Frederick Gutekunst in 1890 with his large-format camera and glass-plate negatives soon gave way to informal, often blurred, snapshots taken by fellow classmates, physicians, nurses, and investigators.

Hopkins has benefited from the efforts of both professional photographers and amateurs—students and residents—over the past century. As students, including Thomas W. Clarke, Murray W. Shulman, Allan Erskine, James E. Mitchell, and J. Michael Criley, photographed their role models, they demonstrated the *esprit de corps* that has characterized Hopkins from its earliest years to the present.

Nationwide, depictions of individual characters and likenesses were not confined to people. The buildings they inhabited, the hospitals or factories in which they worked, the schools and colleges in which they learned, the scenic places they visited—all became subjects for the new generation of Americans who took photographs.

One consequence of the burgeoning popularity of photography was the anonymity of many of the photographers. The absence of this piece of information—the identity of the photographer— eliminates what can be an important contribution to the "truth" of a photograph; furthermore, the usefulness of photographic images, as the historian John Kouwenhoven has pointed out, depends in part upon how much reliable information about them exists.[8]

Some of the photographers in this volume re-main anonymous. Yet this gap in our information about the photographs detracts little from their "truth." Each photograph is but the image of a unique moment, and as such presents only that fragment of history. The changes in the physical spaces at Hopkins may be interpreted as readily from these photographs as the changes in the medical school's curriculum can be reconstructed by the selection and interpretation of a series of curriculum reports. Neither process assures us of truth or completeness. Both enrich our understanding of the past.

As volume I of this centennial history reveals, the development of excellence in American medicine has made Johns Hopkins one among many superior medical institutions. All so-called academic medical centers in this country grew rapidly in the decades after World War II. Similarly, the more recent photographs of medicine at Johns Hopkins have a universal quality, giving the impression that they could have been taken at any leading medical center. The photographs from this more recent era document a changing world of medicine in general, using Hopkins as the exemplar. Just as old photographs assist us in documenting a changing society, so these images help us to describe the changing medical scene in this one institution in a particular American city. Neither the recent pictures, nor the trends, nor the events they portray are unique to Hopkins or to Baltimore. They are shown in order to add to our understanding of American medicine in the last one hundred years and to illustrate the development of one medical institution that became "a model of its kind."

1

THE OPENING OF
THE JOHNS HOPKINS HOSPITAL, 1889

The illustrations in this first section show the beginnings of the Johns Hopkins Hospital, the construction that culminated in the opening of the hospital in 1889. The plans laid out (and revised) by John Shaw Billings appear in this section, along with photographs of the completed hospital buildings and their first occupants.

Most of the photographs of the buildings were taken by Frederick Gutekunst of Philadelphia, whom the trustees hired for this purpose at the opening of the hospital in 1889. Gutekunst was born in Germantown, Pennsylvania, a suburb of Philadelphia, in 1831, and spent his entire life in Philadelphia. When he was engaged by the trustees to photograph the newly completed hospital, he was already well known for his large panorama of the Centennial Exhibition of 1876, and for his portrait of President Ulysses S. Grant. The list of subjects who came to his Arch Street studio reads like a "Who Was Who" of American history.[1]

It may seem inappropriate for the trustees to have chosen one of the premiere portrait photographers in the country to memorialize a group of buildings. Yet what Gutekunst did was to treat each hospital building as a subject and each of his photographs as a portrait.

Gutekunst's photographs of the hospital are technically advanced for the time, and the 1890 volume commemorating the opening of the hospital was one of the earliest collections of such high-quality photographs. Reviewers complained that the illustrations in Jacob Riis's book, *How the Other Half Lives*, also published in 1890, were

murky and unclear.[2] Certainly the Gutekunst photographs could not be criticized on that score.

Yet despite Gutekunst's technical expertise, these photographs are strikingly lifeless—they are largely devoid of people. It is somewhat numbing to look at so many photographs of buildings, especially since the heart of Hopkins has always been people—those who work here and those who come to be healed.

It should be remembered that our buildings and machinery are simply tools and instruments, that the real Hospital, the moving and animating soul of the institution which is to do its work and determine its character, consists of the brains to be put in it.

—John Shaw Billings
letter to trustees, July 1876

Except for his photographs of the Pathology Building, Gutekunst took many of the pictures before the buildings were occupied. As a result, his photographs of the Pathology Building's interiors, showing bottles on the shelves and microscopes on the tables, are slightly warmer and more vivid than many of the others. The quality that all his photographs of the hospital have in common, however, is their concrete representation of the spaces conjured up by the hospital's planners.

From the planning phase that began in the

1870s to the opening of the hospital in 1889 was a very long process. By the time of his death in 1873, Johns Hopkins had not only provided three and one-half million dollars for a university and an equal sum for a hospital, but he had chosen a board of trustees for each and had purchased the property to site his hospital. These trustees—and their appointee, John Shaw Billings—were responsible for the buildings that Gutekunst memorialized.

The line drawings in this section represent the novel ideas of John Shaw Billings, whose extensive role in planning both the hospital and the medical school is not generally appreciated. He was an expert in hospital design and construction, an indefatigable bibliographer, and, in general, a superb organizer. During the years he planned the Johns Hopkins Hospital, Billings was also compiling the massive *Index Catalog* of the Surgeon General's Library, as well as the *Index Medicus*.

In after years, Dr. Billings stated in private conversations that he had prepared two sets of plans, one of which corresponded closely with the usual plan of hospital construction in the United States and England, consisting of a central administration building with wings of two or three stories on either side designed to give about the same accommodations for the sick as were then afforded in other hospitals. Such a building in his estimation would be comparatively inexpensive. His second, or alternative plan, was a lay-out closely resembling the one finally adopted. It provided for a more elaborate administration building (with private wards on either side), a large nurses' home, a kitchen building, and rows of pavilions of one-story, situated above a connecting corridor that permitted free passage beneath the wards to and from the different buildings and gave access to the grounds without passing through the wards themselves. The cost of erecting this second set of plans would unquestionably be considerably greater than the cost of the first set, but Dr. Billings said that when both were presented to the Board of Trustees, it was promptly decided to adopt the second or pavilion plan.

—Henry M. Hurd
First Superintendent of the Hospital[3]

The pavilion plan for hospital design was favored by Florence Nightingale and others, who believed that such construction afforded a maximum of fresh air and sunshine, hence minimizing the much-dreaded spread of infection.[4]

Even with the most perfect arrangement it is impossible to secure absolute immunity. An incident within my own knowledge will exhibit the potency of the cause of contamination and the facility of diffusion.

A passer on the street heard a tap at a window, and, pausing, it was thrown up, and a gentleman, seated within, said: "Are you afraid of varioloid?" The passer replied: "Yes, but draw down the sash and I will talk to you." It was done immediately, yet in due time to prove the source of poisoning, he sickened with the disease. This was lateral diffusion; and while it shows the subtle nature of the miasm, and the necessity for adopting every guard against it, proves that all that can be done is ineffectual to annihilate the influence.

—Caspar Morris[5]

The opening of the hospital at last enabled William Osler, William S. Halsted, and Howard A. Kelly to begin their work at Hopkins. William H. Welch, the guiding spirit of Hopkins, had already moved into his laboratory on the hospital grounds. It was largely through the efforts of these four leaders of medicine at Johns Hopkins that the hospital thrived in its early years.

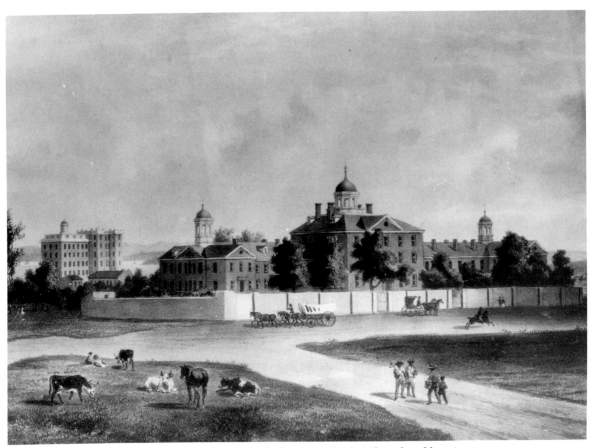

This undated print shows the Maryland Hospital for the Insane on the site of Loudenschlager's Hill. Mr. Hopkins purchased the land in 1872 when this hospital was moved to its Spring Grove location in Catonsville. The following year, he turned the deed over to his trustees. The purchase price was $150,000 for the tract of about thirteen acres, bounded by Wolfe, Monument, Broadway, and Jefferson streets. The fresh breezes blowing across the slightly elevated site were thought by the hospital planners to be important in reducing the spread of contagious disease from and to the hospital.

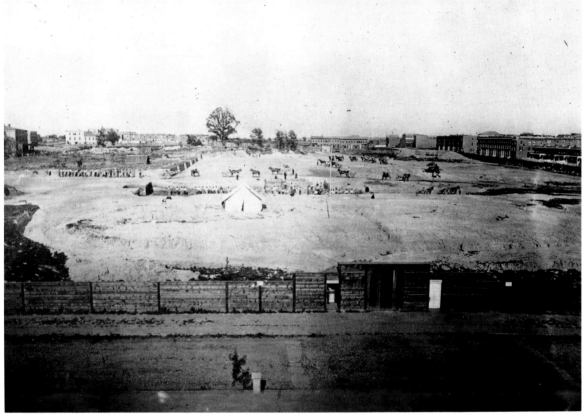

The site purchased from the Maryland State Hospital was cleared soon after that hospital was moved to Catonsville. This photograph, which probably dates from about 1877, shows the land cleared and prepared for construction of the Johns Hopkins Hospital. The small tent in the center of the photograph was the headquarters for the construction supervisor.

By the end of the year 1877, excavations for the cellars of the main building, pay ward and nurses' home had been completed; the lot had been drained, the foundations laid, and the walls of the principal buildings begun. Sketches for the elevation of the main building and pay wards forming the west front of the Hospital were prepared by Cabot and Chandler of Boston and were approved by the Trustees. The style of architecture adopted was Queen Anne, the material brick, with trimmings of dark blue Cheat River stone. On February 12, 1878, Dr. Billings presented his final report on the system of heating and ventilation, which, as he remarked, was specially designed for the climate of Baltimore and the location and lay-out of the Hospital.

—Henry M. Hurd[6]

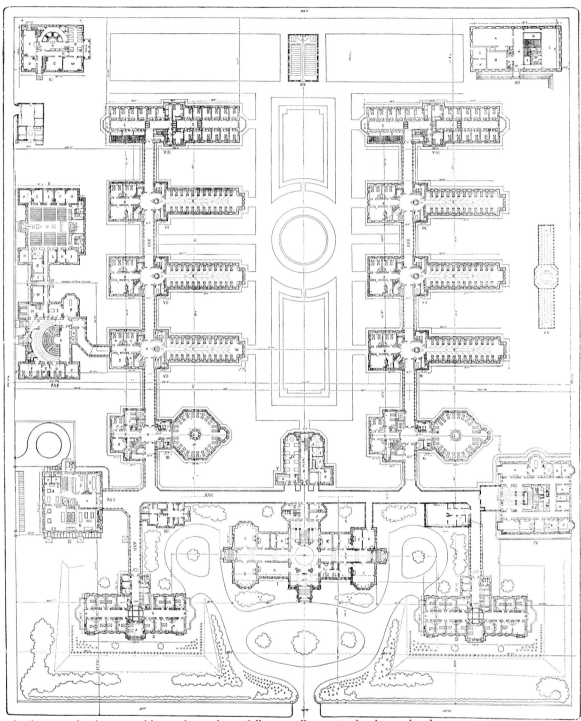

The drawings for the original hospital were beautifully, as well as meticulously, rendered. Unlike so many American universities and hospitals, this one grew initially according to a set of carefully crafted plans.

In the original block plan, the Administration Building appears in the center, flanked by the Male and Female Pay Wards (the wards for private patients). The Dispensary and Amphitheater were located just to the north of the Common Wards. (A "block plan" is a detailed line drawing, less complex than a blueprint or architect's rendering.)

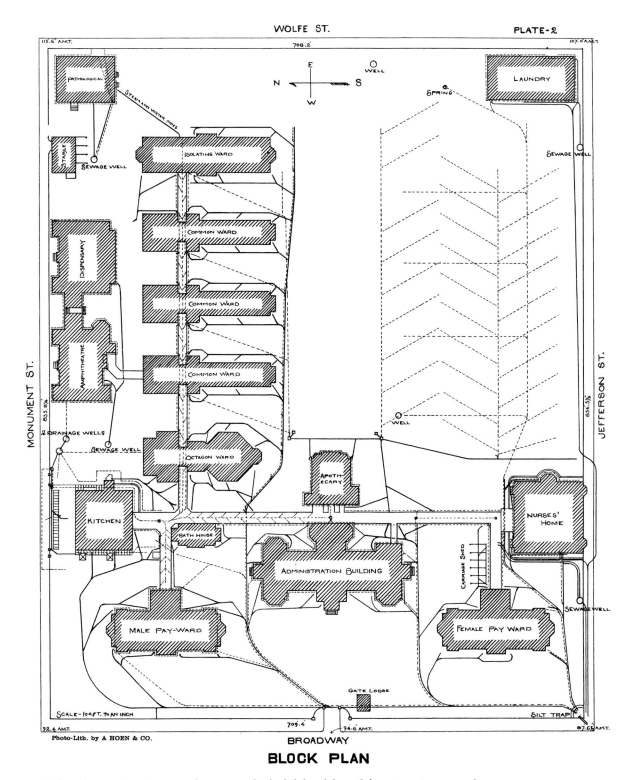

BLOCK PLAN

In the subsequent construction, however, only the left-hand face of the mirror-image wards was completed, owing to a lack of funds. This later block plan, which shows what was actually built, reveals the striking absence of symmetry in the lines of ward buildings.

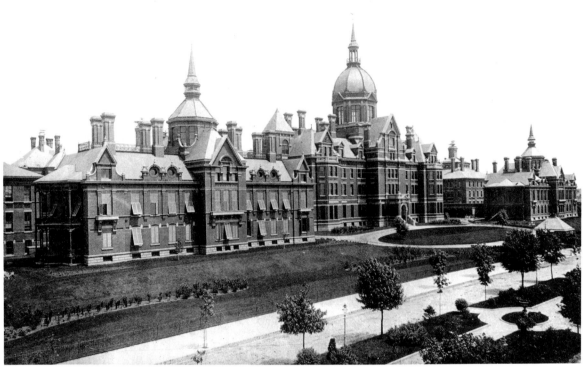

One of Frederick Gutekunst's photographs of the hospital, taken from Broadway looking south-east. Before it was torn down in 1963, the gatehouse (shown in closeup on the facing page) served for a time as a gift shop.

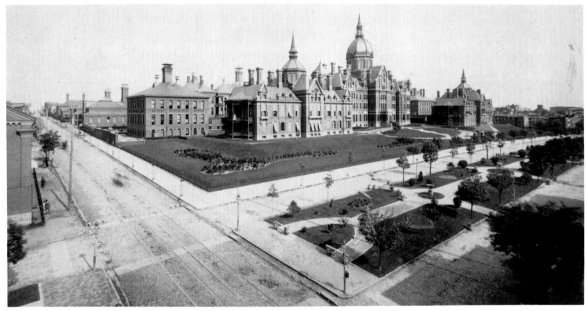

A similar view revealing Monument Street running along the left (north) side of the hospital buildings. Closest to Monument Street on the main hospital grounds was the kitchen building, which also contained the heating plant. The building on the far right is the Nurses' Home. Broadway is seen as a divided street, a century-old characteristic that it has retained.

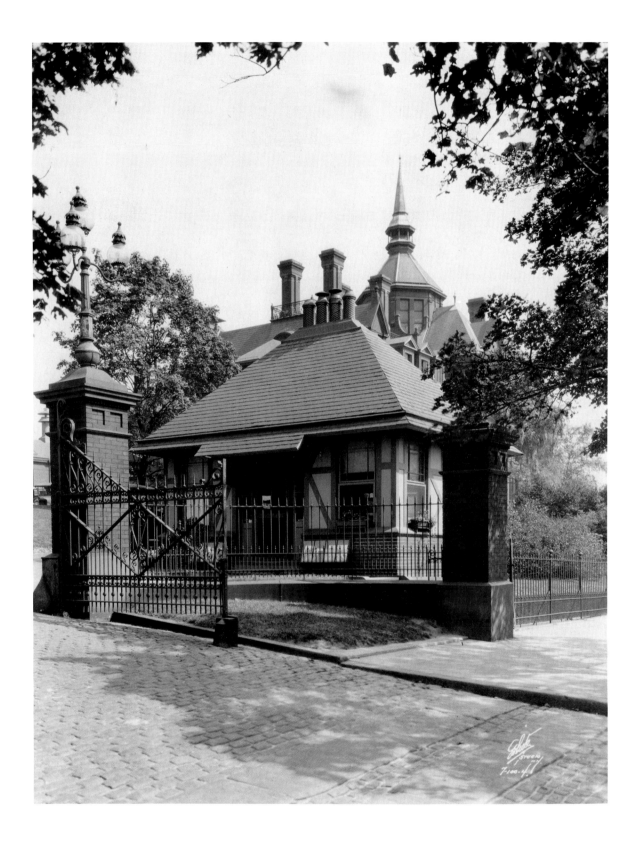

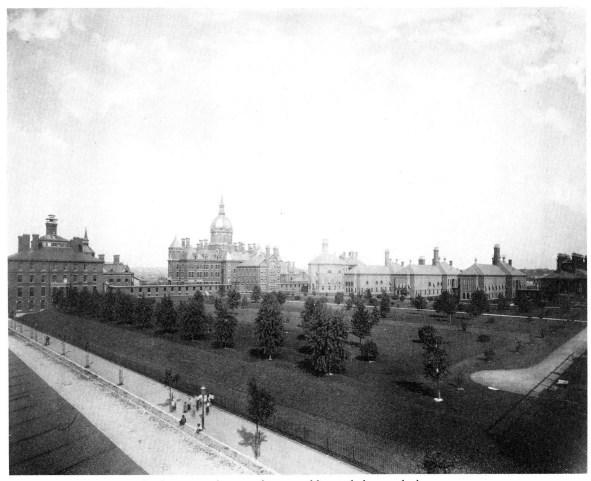

This photograph illustrates the discrepancy between the original hospital plans and what was eventually constructed.

The rear view of the building and grounds was taken from the southeast. The three Common Wards, for nonpaying patients, are on the right. The Octagon Ward, later named the Thayer Building, is located between the Common Wards and the Administration Building.

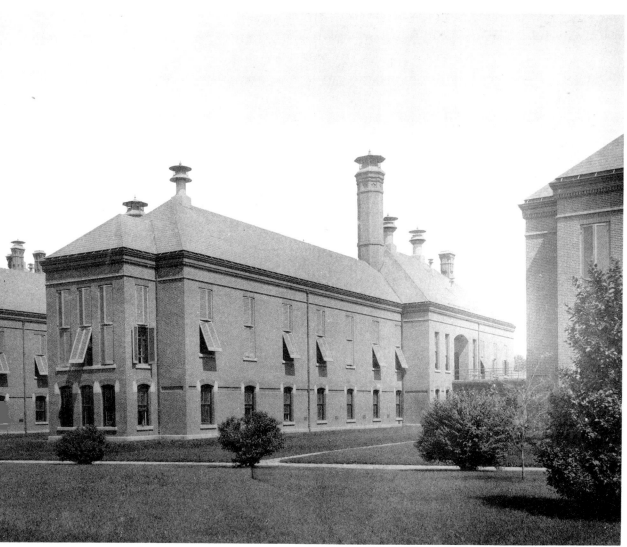

The Common Wards were two stories, a ground floor on the level with the connecting corridor, and a main floor, level with the bridge, as shown at the right of the exterior view. These buildings had no elevators, so patients had to be transported up and down by stretcher.

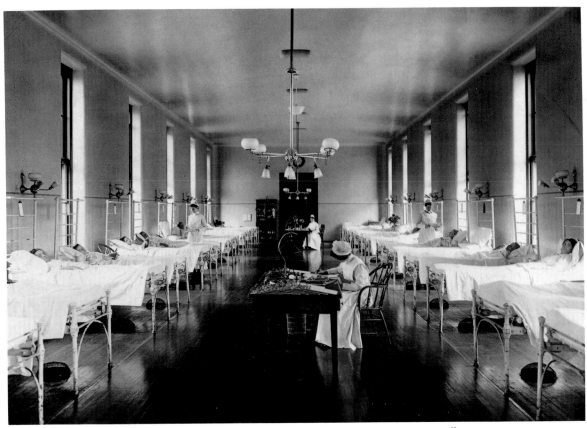

There was no running water in the wards, and as shown in the private room, patients as well as staff used washbowls. Note, too, the ventilators on the floor under each bed, which could be individually regulated to provide fresh air.

The interior of each Common Ward contained twelve beds on each side. Windows were abundant, but there was no provision for any privacy. Natural light from the windows was augmented by lighting from gas fixtures, although Billings had prudently suggested that electric wiring be introduced in the original construction, since the day of electric light was at hand. The gas fixtures were especially designed for the hospital: they were simple and rounded to afford easy cleaning.

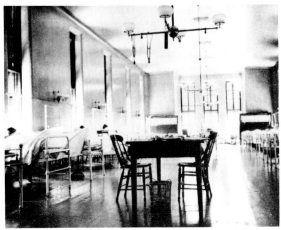

Note the stethoscopes suspended from the gaslights.

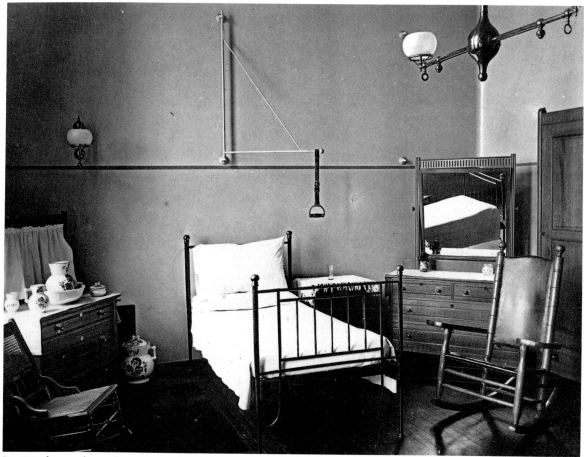

Pay Wards were located on either side and in front of the Administration Building. This view shows a hospital room that was relatively comfortable for the time, despite the absence of rug and wall decoration. Note the washbowl and chamber pot. Toilets were at the end of the corridor.

Another peculiarity of the sick wards is the arrangement for easy cleansing, and to prevent possible accumulations of dust in corners and crevices. Corners are to a great extent done away with, and easy curves given in their place; even at the junction of the floor and walls there is a curve instead of the usual right angle, and I advise you to look at it and see how it has been produced, for it ought to become fashionable, and take the place of the old mop-board in all well-constructed houses.

—John Shaw Billings
Address, Opening Day of
The Johns Hopkins Hospital
May 7, 1889[7]

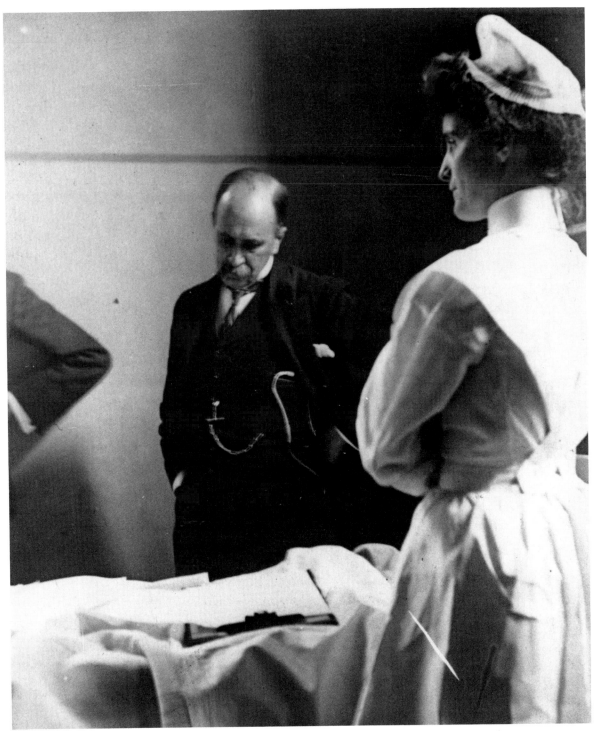

The first physician-in-chief of the Johns Hopkins Hospital was William Osler. Osler was a clinician and a teacher, and it is in these capacities that we see him here. He taught by both the spoken and the written word, and by the force of his personality.

   These well-known snapshots of Osler at the bedside show him engaging in the clinical tasks of observing, palpating, auscultating, and contemplating. They were taken by Thomas W. Clarke, a graduate of the school of medicine in the Class of 1902.

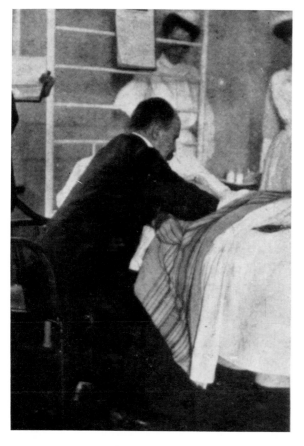

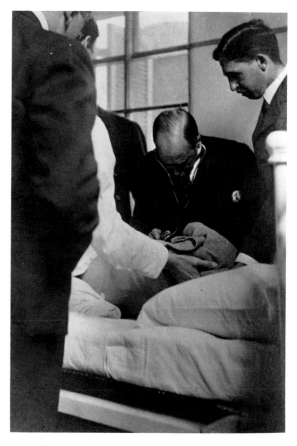

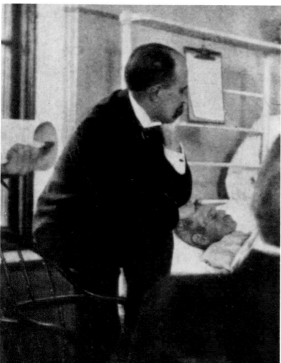

I wish to tell a plain tale of the method of teaching medicine at The Johns Hopkins University. There is nothing very novel about it, except that in the third and fourth years the hospital is made the equivalent of the laboratories of the first and second; and in it the student learns the practical art of medicine. This may be called the natural mode of teaching the subject.

It is in the ward, after all, that the student must learn to recognize and to treat disease.

The graduate of a quarter of a century ago went out with little practical knowledge, which increased only as his practice increased. In the natural method of teaching the student begins with the patient, continues with the patient, and ends his studies with the patient, using books and lectures as tools, as means to an end.

—William Osler[8]

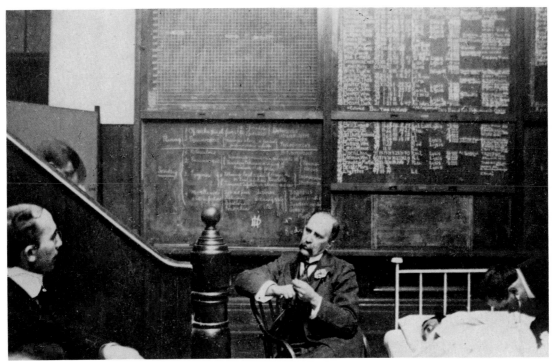

In his many essays, Osler hoped to inspire a love of learning and of books. In his classic article, "The Natural Method of Teaching the Subject of Medicine," published in the Journal of the American Medical Association, he left for posterity the precepts by which he instructed students and residents at the Johns Hopkins Hospital.

This photograph shows Osler conducting a clinic in the Amphitheater ca. 1900.

That the medical student is an essential factor in the life of a great general hospital, has been of slow recognition in this country. Admitted to the dispensaries, welcomed in the amphitheater, he has been, until recently, rigidly excluded from the wards, except as a casual attendant on ward classes. I am glad to say that from the day he leaves the medical school laboratories, he is in this hospital a co-worker with doctors and nurses, in every one of its activities, and as his right, not as a privilege grudgingly granted by the trustees.

—William Osler[9]

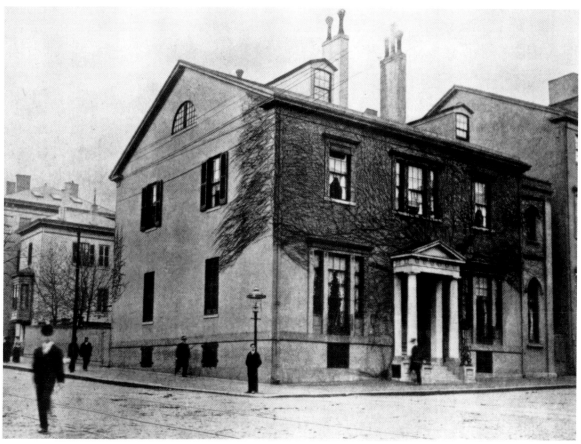

After Osler's marriage to Grace Revere Gross in 1892, students and residents were often in-vited to their home at the corner of West Franklin and Charles streets in downtown Baltimore. Those who were given keys—Harvey Cushing, Thomas B. Futcher, and Henry Barton Jacobs—were called the "Latchkeyers" and lived next door at 3 West Franklin, at the right of the photograph.

I have always felt that in his third-year clinic Dr. Osler reached the high-water-mark of clini-cal teaching—that indeed he here spoke the last word in the teaching art. This was not the con-ventional clinic—a lecture or demonstration. In-stead he became one of a group of students, none of whom except himself had any knowledge of disease except that acquired from the study of dead tissues. Together they observed and de-scribed sick human beings. The special examples studied he himself had not previously seen, but they were chosen at random by his assistants from among those applying for treatment. One student was chosen to conduct the examination under Dr. Osler's direction, though each of the members of the class quickly became as inter-ested and keen as though he were personally making the examination. By skilful direction the students were guided in detecting the particular features in which the patient differed from the normal. Dr. Osler looked and the students looked with him. Then they were guided in reasoning from effect to cause and cause to effect.

—Rufus I. Cole[10]

Once the hospital had opened for patients, residents were a constant presence on the wards.
Ward rounds by residents and staff physicians have been a familiar feature since the beginning.

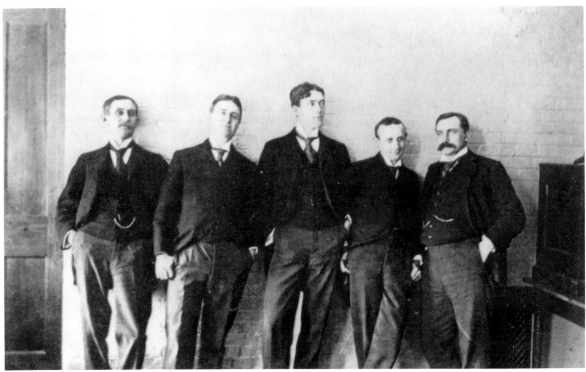

These early residents and fellows, shown ca. 1891, worked with Welch or Osler. Note their
dress, the similarity of which, though probably unintentional, was the "uniform" of the day.
(Left to right: Franklin P. Mall, William S. Thayer, Lewellys F. Barker, Simon Flexner, and
Frank R. Smith.)

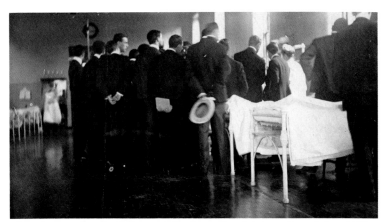

This photograph, which shows medical rounds, also dates from before 1921,
the year in which residents began to wear white uniforms.

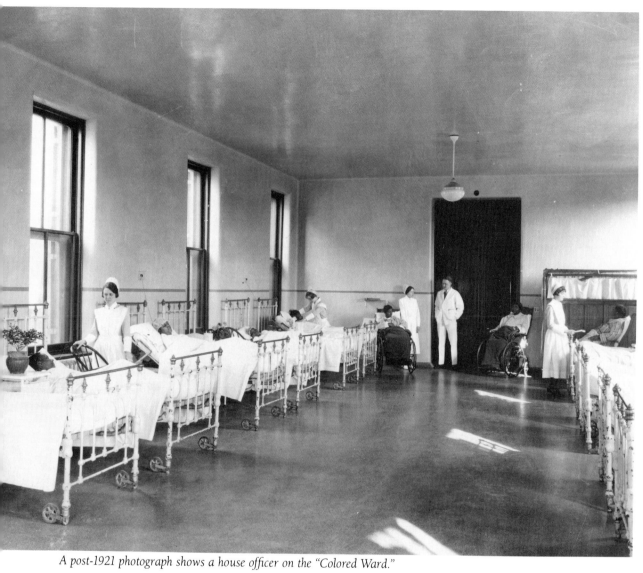

A post-1921 photograph shows a house officer on the "Colored Ward."

Osler and Thayer were men of entirely different personalities. Osler's power was that of inspiration; Thayer's, response to inspiration. Osler was a leader; Thayer, a keen-sighted independent follower of the leaders in his profession. As Thayer worked in the Hospital and caught light from the world's great medical sources, he turned that light always on them, not on himself, unaware of his own striking individuality and the quality that was uniquely his own. Few have done more than he to keep the achievements of great physicians before the world.

—Edith Gittings Reid[11]

[M]edicine, what a wonderful opportunity it offered! Based on the fundamental sciences for the aid of which it was reaching out more and more every day, what a fascinating problem the art of medicine! What curious misapprehensions had been his! How little had he grasped the significance of the human side of medicine! What a childish, ridiculous thought that medicine could be practised by rigid rules; that the day was near when we could seek the answer to every diagnostic problem by a chemical reaction; that we could treat our patients by rule of thumb! What an absurd fancy that all the physiological and chemical and physical knowledge in the world could give one the art of Fowler [Osler] without laborious study and practice at the bedside and in association with human beings. And what an immense reward to gain in the end— something of the deftness of touch, the keenness of vision, the sureness of judgement which only experience can give!

—William S. Thayer
"The Medical Education of Jones"

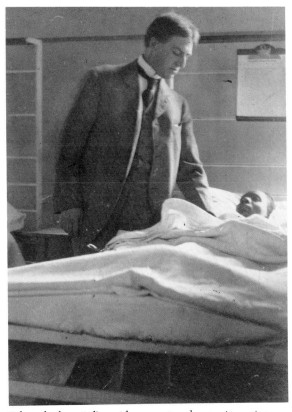

When the hospital's residency system began, its major purpose was to train masters who would carry on the precepts of the Hopkins model. William S. Thayer, who was Osler's resident physician from 1891 to 1898, was an outstanding example of the concept's success. He became professor of medicine in 1919, and brought outstanding young scientists such as Alphonse R. Dochez, Walter W. Palmer, Dana W. Atchley, and Robert F. Loeb to the Department of Medicine.

Osler's "natural method of teaching" was followed by his successors, each of whom imparted his own personal style to instruction on rounds. These masters thus provided a variety of role models for students and house staff.

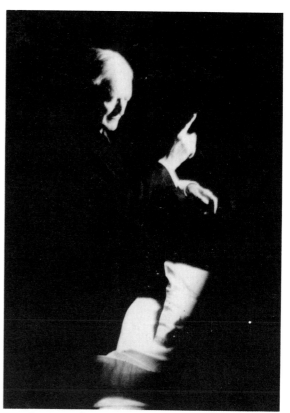

Lewellys F. Barker

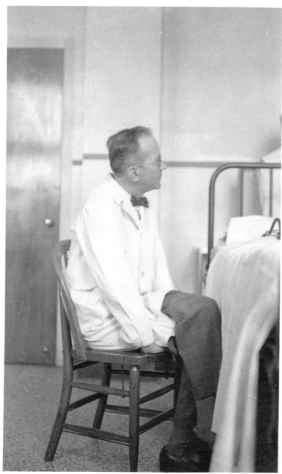

Louis Hamman

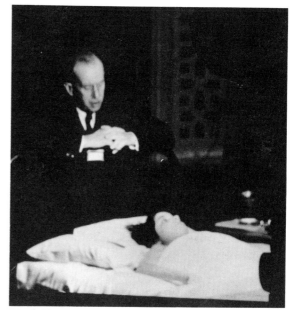

Warfield T. Longcope.

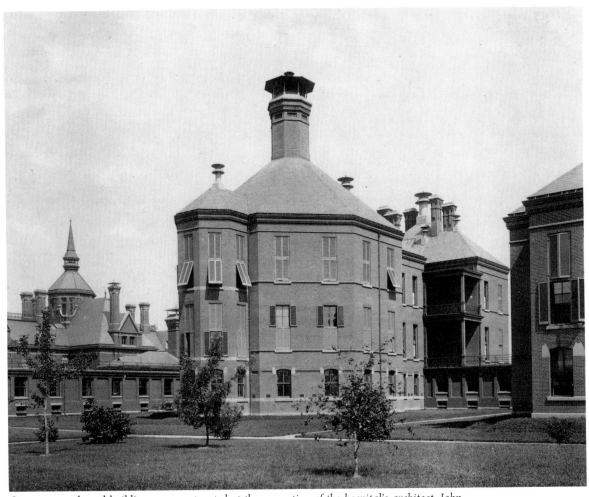

One octagon-shaped building was constructed at the suggestion of the hospital's architect, John Niernsee. He believed that a square or octagonal shape afforded the best exposure to sunlight and the most even distribution of heat. The other argument for its use was that it provided the largest area per bed for the lowest cost in space and money. In contrast to the other wards, the Octagon Ward had three floors instead of two.

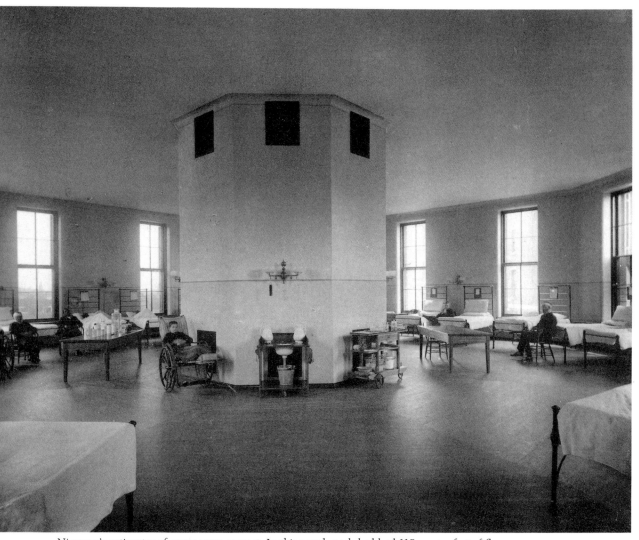

Niernsee's estimates of space were correct. In this ward, each bed had 115 square feet of floor space, as opposed to 107 square feet in the Common Wards. (It is hard to say whether this difference was significant from the patient's point of view.) In both this and the Common Ward, one side of every bed was near a window. The long windows afforded maximum daylight—an important feature, as the gas lights provided relatively little illumination.

As is evident from the patients with their bandages, the Octagon Ward was used for surgical as well as medical patients.

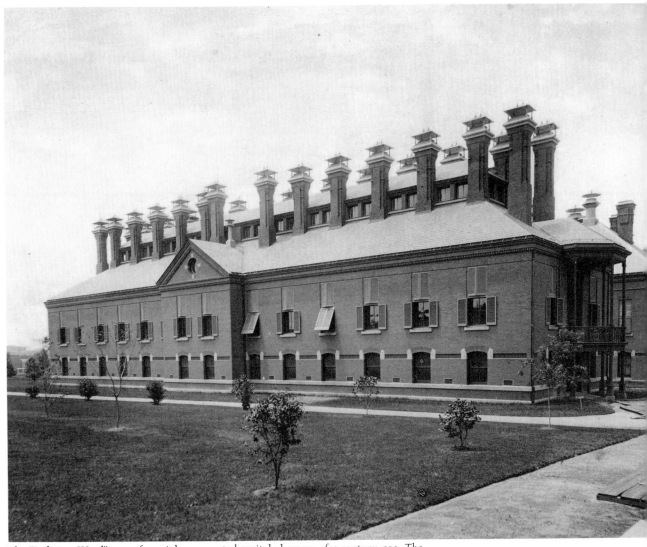

The "Isolating Ward" was of special concern to hospital planners of a century ago. The mid-1870s was nearly a decade after Joseph Lister had extended Pasteur's theories of germs in the air, but the so-called golden age of bacteriology began in 1876 with Robert Koch's demonstration of the anthrax bacillus. When the Johns Hopkins Hospital was built, therefore, the knowledge that disease spreads through the air was well established.

This building, seen here from the northeast, was located at the extreme end of the hospital's main east-west corridor, where the Meyer Building is today. The ward consisted of twenty private rooms for patients, each with its own ventilation and chimney, and accommodation for four nurses, who lived in the ward for about one week at a time. While on duty, the nurses were required to remain on the ward to minimize the spread of infection.

As Billings noted, all the rooms opened to a corridor "through which the wind is always blowing." Billings and the architects went to great lengths to prevent the spread of contagion. The walls were of double thickness. In some of the rooms, air came from the basement in a constant, one-way flow. Thus, no one rebreathed the air, and the effect was that of being out of doors in a gentle breeze.

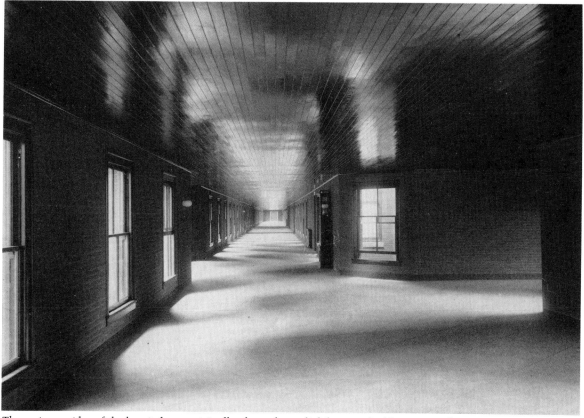

The main corridor of the hospital was originally planned as a link between buildings or pavilions. This corridor has been a distinctive feature of the hospital throughout its history. Despite many changes and additions to the configuration and arrangements of the buildings, the corridors have linked the people, the buildings, and the years. Hundreds of thousands of people have traversed these corridors in the past century, and they hold a permanent place in the memories of all who have studied and worked at Johns Hopkins.

This photograph shows the main corridor as photographed by Gutekunst in 1889.

The Long Corridor, linking the years as well as the buildings themselves, extends for a quarter mile or more, its eastern end open to Wolfe Street and the School of Hygiene, its southern end reaching the Wilmer Clinic and the new Oncology Center, passing on the way most of the other Hopkins buildings. Its doors were not locked for 90 years. Rarely empty day or night, the Long Corridor in its ever-changing whirl of humanity reflects the purposefulness, grimness, gaiety, and bustle of the mixture of staff, patients, and visitors.

—Thomas B. Turner
Dean, The Johns Hopkins University
School of Medicine, 1957–68[12]

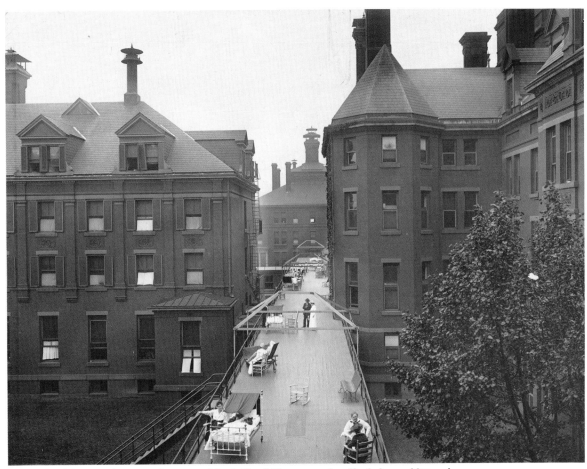

The roofs of the corridors were known as "the Bridge." They not only afforded an additional walkway, but as seen here, they were used to bring patients into fresh air and sunshine.

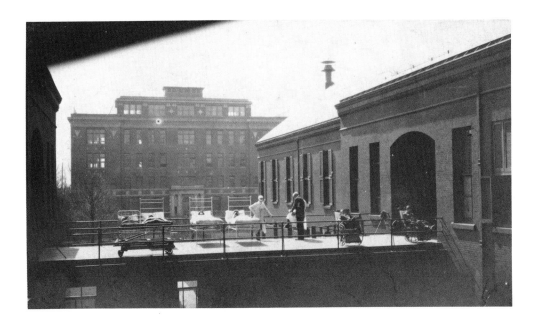

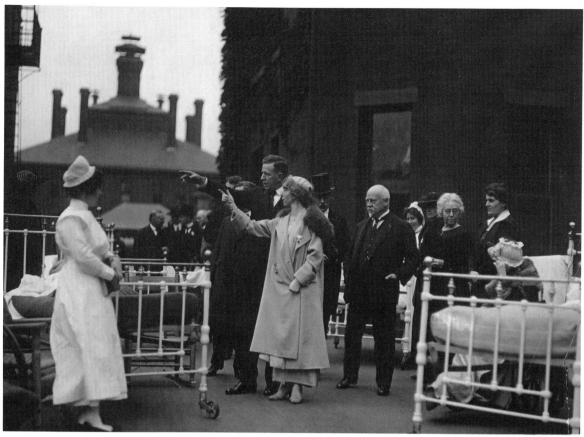

The Bridge was also a feature of the tour given the Queen and King of Belgium on their visit to the hospital in 1919. Welch and Hospital Superintendent Winford Smith, along with University President Frank J. Goodnow, are seen guiding the royal visitors.

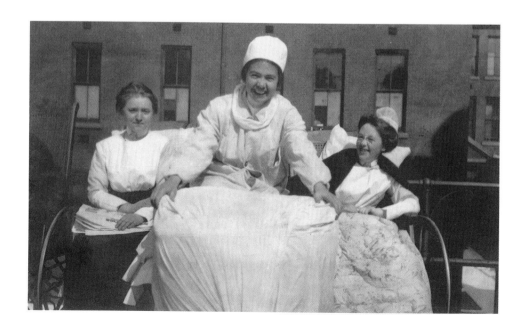

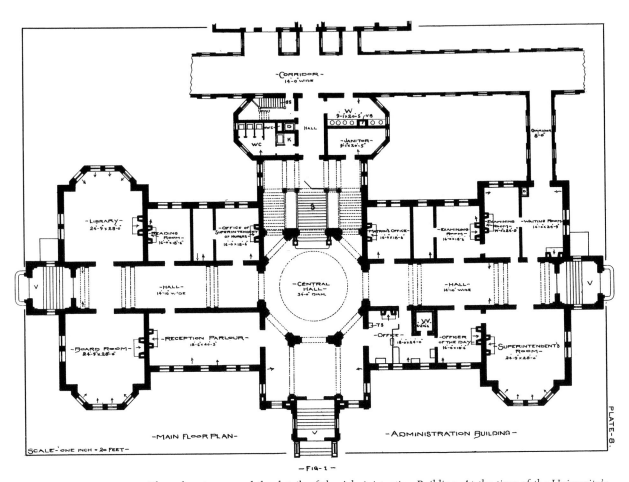

-FIG-1-

These drawings reveal the details of the Administration Building. At the time of the University's centennial in 1976, this building was officially named the John Shaw Billings Building, and it was added to the National Register of Historic Buildings.

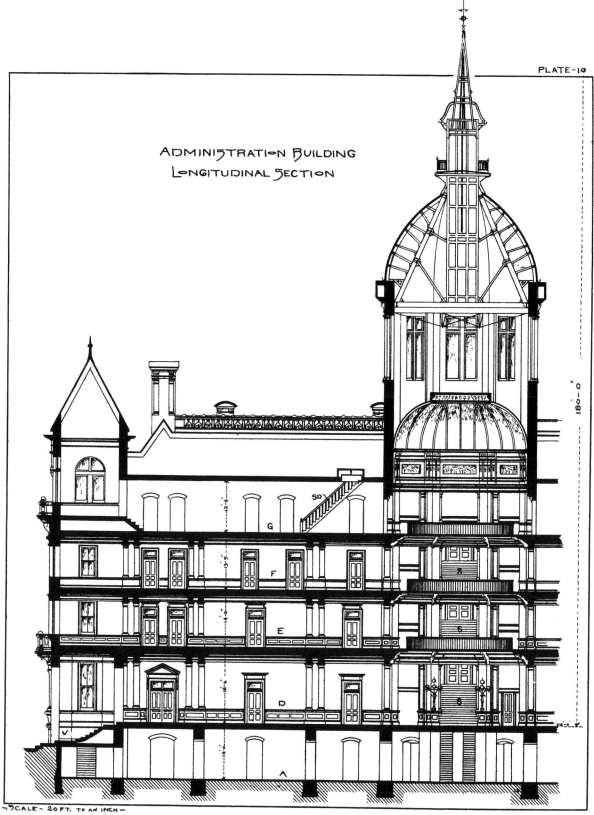

ADMINISTRATION BUILDING
LONGITUDINAL SECTION

PLATE-10

180-0"

-SCALE- 20 FT. TO AN INCH-

-FIG. 1-

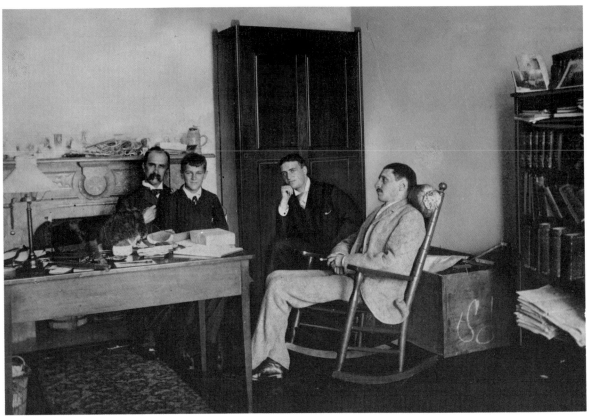

Generations of house officers lived on the upper floors from the hospital's opening until the 1950s. This photograph, taken in Henri LaFleur's room in 1891, shows Osler with his first two residents. LaFleur (in the rocker) was packing for his return to Montreal; William S. Thayer, in the middle, replaced him as resident that year. Sitting on Osler's lap is his nephew W. W. Francis, who seems to be looking at the cat on the table. (Francis became a graduate of the medical school Class of 1903.) Note the battered top hat, which they had used as a football, on the table.

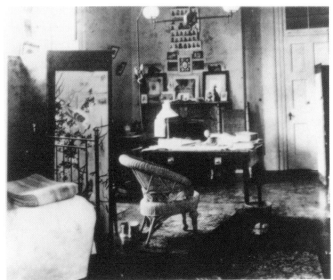

A typical room "under the Dome."

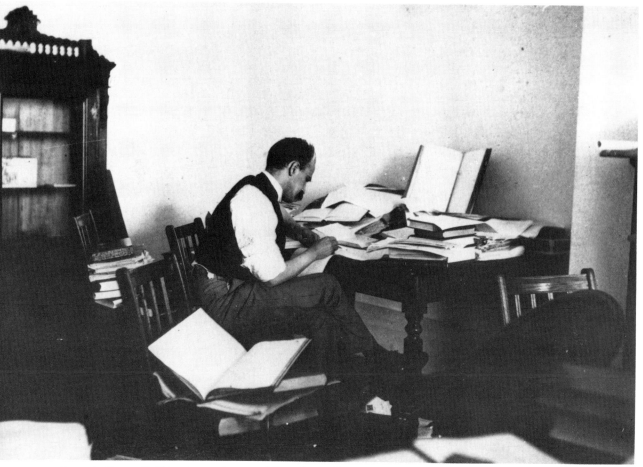

It was in Hunter Robb's suite on the second floor that William Osler wrote his influential text-book of medicine. (Hunter Robb was the first resident in gynecology.)

He asked me if I would loan him the use of my library for an hour or so in the mornings. I of course said, "Yes, with great pleasure." The first morning, he appeared with one book under his arm accompanied by his stenographer, Miss Humpton. When the morning's work was over, he left the book on my library desk, wide open with a marker in it. The next morning he brought two books with him, and so on for the next two weeks, so that the table and all the chairs and the sofa and the piano and even the floor was covered with open books. As a consequence I never was able to use the room for fully six months. Oftentimes right in the middle of his dictating he would stop and rush into my other room, and ask me to match quarters with him, or we would engage in an exchange of yarns. It was a great treat for me, and except when he could court inspiration by kicking my waste-paper basket about the room, I thoroughly enjoyed his visits.

—Hunter Robb[13]

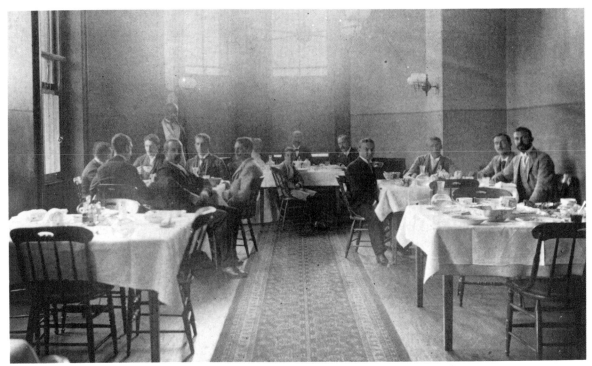

The staff dining room (shown here ca. 1890) was an important meeting place for the early faculty and their residents.

At first, with the exception of Welch and Mall, we all lived in the hospital, our rooms in the main building were capacious, comfortably furnished, and the outlook over the city and harbour was fine. No one of the small group of men who participated in the hospital life at this early period can forget its fascination. . . . We breakfasted together, then each sought his particular duties, to meet again at luncheon. The luncheon hour, at which most of those working at the hospital gathered, was the most delightful of the day. Osler, Welch, Halsted, Mall, LaFleur, and with the usual visiting stranger, sat at a table in the end of the diningroom. The conversation was always lively and interesting: everyone sought to bring something to the feast.

—William T. Councilman[14]

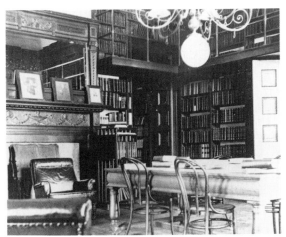

The hospital library was housed in the Administration Building. It was a major reference source until the Welch Medical Library was opened in 1929.

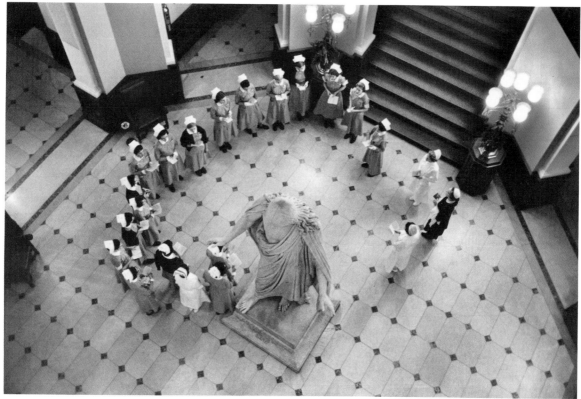

In 1896, a copy of the statue of Christ by the Danish sculptor Thorwaldsen was placed in the rotunda of the Administration Building, under the dome.

We are assembled in the presence of one of the best works of modern Christian sculpture,—a transcendent theme, treated by an illustrious art-ist, in his noblest manner; a work, too that has stood the test of more than seventy-five years without a word of censorious criticism. Canova saw it in Rome, while it was modeling by the artist and praised it. The people of Copenhagen determined to have it. It was reproduced at Postdam (Berlin) in front of the Church of Peace, near which the Emperor Frederic lies buried. A copy, in plaster, surrounded by the twelve apos-tles, from the same artist, was brought to New York at least forty years ago and exhibited in what was known as the Crystal Palace or the World's Fair.

—Daniel C. Gilman[15]

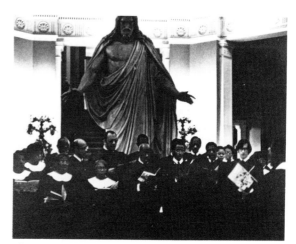

This photograph shows the Memorial Baptist Church Choir giving its annual Christmas concert in the ro-tunda. The singing of carols began in the rotunda. The choir, followed by a group of physicians and nurses, would then visit each ward in turn.

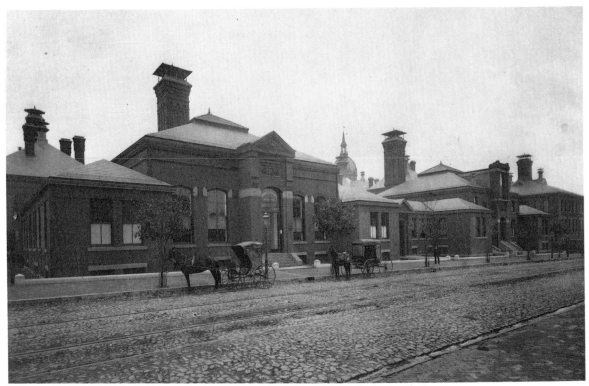

The Dispensary and Amphitheater were located in a one-story building on the south side of Monument Street, where the Carnegie Building now stands. They were thus close to the land owned by the University where the medical school buildings would soon be constructed.

The large Amphitheater, shown in a Gutekunst photograph at upper right, had seats for 280. Next door was an operating room with a large bay window for good light, an anesthesia room, a recovery room, a room for surgeons, a three-bed ward for postoperative patients, and an accident room with two beds.

The Dispensary had seating for 400, but on a hot day, the wait must have been difficult. Medicines were dispensed from the pharmacy on the south side of the waiting room.

The care of ambulatory patients, a vital part of the hospital at its founding, has become increasingly important at the start of Hopkins' second century. In the late nineteenth century, when the hospital was built, hospital facilities for outpatients were unusual, as patients were cared for either at home or in their physician's office. Billings emphasized the importance of the Dispensary to the clinical mission of the hospital. Osler implemented the important role of the Dispensary in the teaching of medical students.

This dispensary is a very important part of the Hospital organization, and may be made the means of doing a much greater amount of good than such institutions usually effect. Through it the majority of the Hospital patients will probably be selected.

—John Shaw Billings[16]

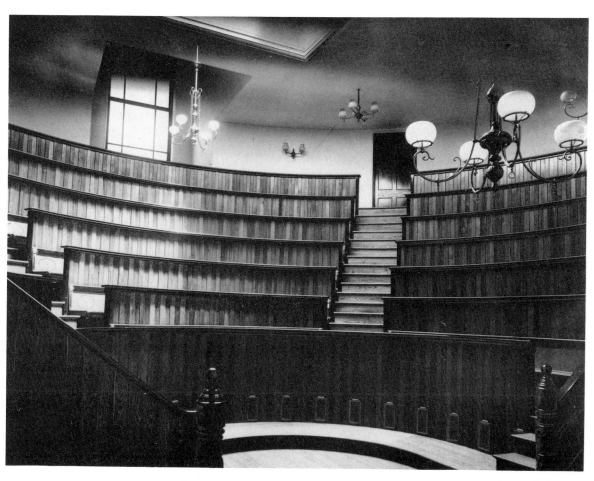

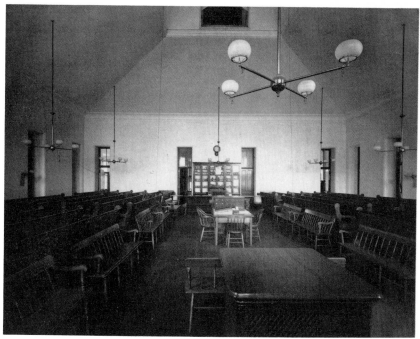

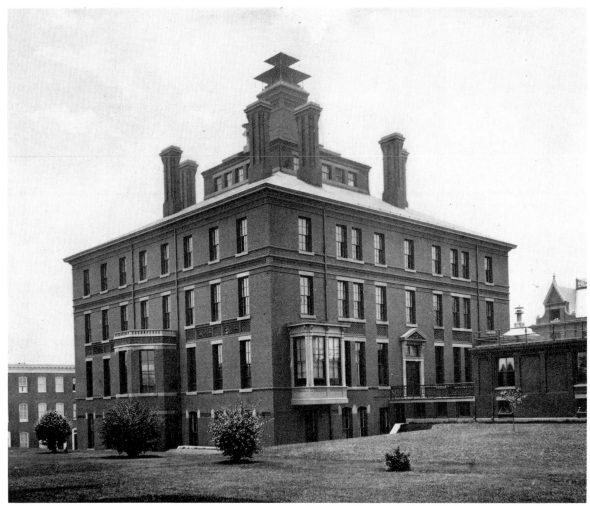

The Nurses' Home was a handsome, square building, situated at the south end of the hospital's north-south corridor, where the Wilmer Institute stands today. The residence for nurses and nursing students was designed for the comfort of its occupants—an indication that the founders of the hospital valued the contribution of nurses.

I can only say that in many cases a competent trained nurse is as important to the success of treatment as a competent doctor, and that one of the greatest difficulties in treating well-to-do patients in their own homes in this city is the want of proper nurses.

—John Shaw Billings[17]

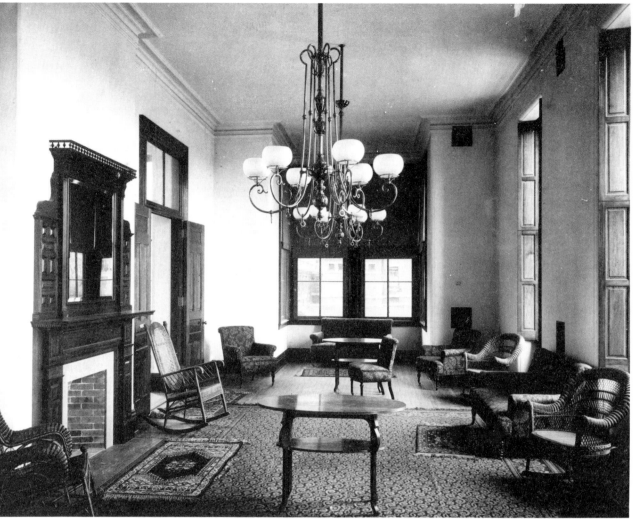

To Billings, the residence for nurses resembled a "well-finished hotel of medium size," and each occupant had a front room that was generously lighted and separately ventilated. Presiding over the nurses' residence was the first superintendent of nurses and head of the Nurses' Training School, Isabel Hampton.

Life in the training school was cheerful and simple. It was Miss Hampton's custom to read prayers just after breakfast, in the parlor, and with military discipline every nurse attended. It was always a new sensation to see her, serene and beautiful, enter the room with her prayer book in hand after the whole staff had taken its place and this impression was not lessened when I learned later that she sometimes dressed in

three and a half minutes. We had a hymn which I played on the piano, then it was our custom to go with the nurses to the door and watch them go down the corridor. . . . Almost always, as we turned away, she would say to me with perhaps a little squeeze of the hands, "Docky, aren't they nice."

—Lavinia Dock
Asst. superintendent of nurses[18]

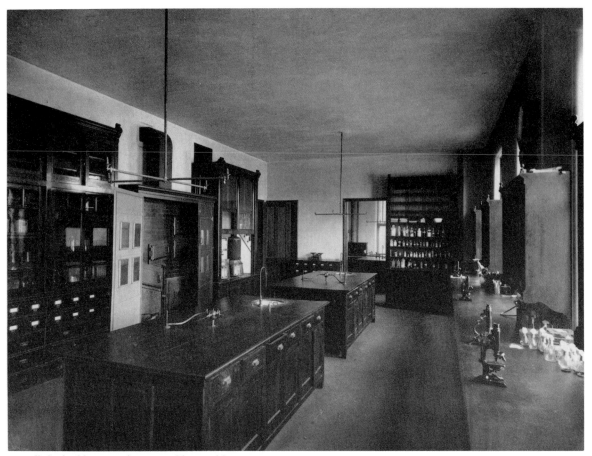

Not all the buildings on the original hospital lot were constructed for the direct (or indirect) care of patients. The Pathology Building, on the northeast corner of the hospital lot, housed Welch's Pathological Laboratory, where young medical scientists came to do research under the general guidance of the first full-time member of the medical faculty brought to Baltimore, William Henry Welch. Here men of the caliber of Simon Flexner and Walter Reed worked, and two future faculty stalwarts, William S. Halsted and Franklin P. Mall, began their Baltimore careers in this building.

It was Welch, after his arrival in Baltimore in 1884, who persuaded the Trustees and the builders of the important connection between the pathology department, which at the time also included bacteriology, and the work of the hospital. By the fall of 1886, Welch and some of his fellows had moved into the two-story building. They had already begun teaching courses on infectious diseases for practicing physicians. Many of these early postgraduate students went on to successful careers, and five of them eventually joined the faculty of the school of medicine, which would open in 1893.

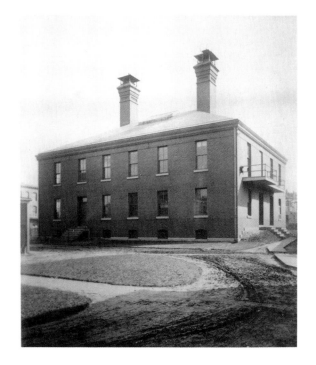

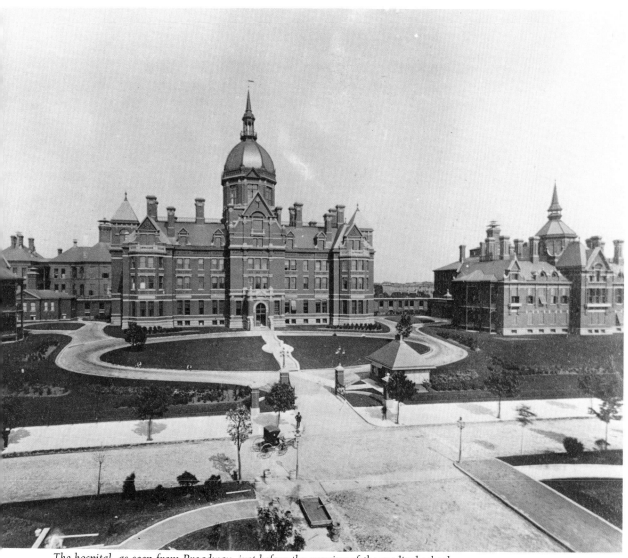

The hospital, as seen from Broadway, just before the opening of the medical school.

2

THE EARLY YEARS OF
THE JOHNS HOPKINS UNIVERSITY
SCHOOL OF MEDICINE, 1893–1914

Section 2 depicts the long-awaited opening of the Johns Hopkins University School of Medicine in 1893, describing in words and pictures some of the events of its early years. William H. Welch had characterized the Johns Hopkins Hospital as "the clinical laboratory of the medical school." Now preclinical laboratories would join the hospital buildings in East Baltimore.

With the opening of the medical school, Johns Hopkins' plan was at last fulfilled. As he had stipulated to his trustees,

> In all your arrangements in relation to this hospital, you will bear constantly in mind that it is my wish and purpose that the institution should ultimately form a part of the medical school of that university for which I have made ample provision by my will.[1]

The medical school's first catalog was a nondescript pamphlet—fifteen pages of plain, gray-brown paper—but it contained a fresh and important document: the text of a speech delivered by Dr. Welch at the graduation exercise of the University in June 1893. Here Welch set forth the philosophy of the new medical school, which has come to be known as the "Hopkins model":

> The aim of the School will be primarily to train practitioners of medicine and surgery, that is to qualify persons to take care of diseased and injured conditions of the human body. We hold that the medical art should rest upon a thorough training in the medical sciences, and that, other things being equal, he is the best practitioner who has this thorough training. The medical sciences have made great progress in the last quarter of a century, greater than has the practice of medicine with which alone the general public has much concern. . . .
>
> But medical education is not completed at the medical school; it is only begun. Hence it is not only or chiefly the quantity of knowledge which the student takes with him from the school which will help him in his future work; it is also the quality of mind, the methods of work, the disciplined habit of correct reasoning, the way of looking at medical problems.
>
> In order to cultivate in the student this habit of thought, this method of work, I believe that there is no one thing so essential as that the teacher should be also an investigator and should be capable of imparting something of the spirit of investigation to the student. The medical school should be a place where medicine is not only taught but also studied. It should do its part to advance medical science and art by encouraging original work, and by selecting as its teachers those who have the training and capacity for such work. In no other department of natural science are to be found problems awaiting solution more attractive, more significant than those in medicine; and certainly these problems do not lose in dignity because they relate to the physical well-being of mankind.
>
> The Johns Hopkins Medical School will start unhampered by traditions and free to work out its own salvation. It will derive inestimable advantage from being an integral and coordinate part of this great University which will see to it that university ideals and methods are not lost sight of in the new school.[2]

The Johns Hopkins Hospital Bulletin.

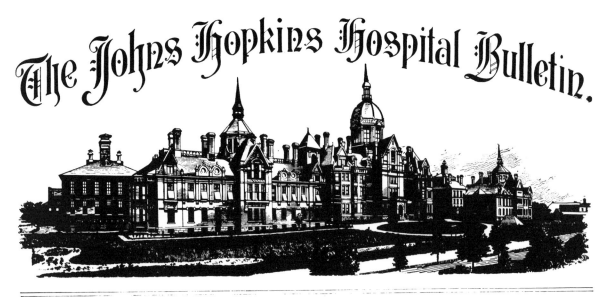

Volume I.—No. 1.]   BALTIMORE, DECEMBER, 1889.   [Price, 15 Cents.

MEDICAL INSTRUCTION IN THE JOHNS HOPKINS HOSPITAL.

During the year 1889–90, instruction will be given at the Johns Hopkins Hospital in Pathology and Bacteriology, Medicine, Surgery, Gynaecology, and Hygiene, by lectures, demonstrations, laboratory courses, bed-side teaching and general clinics in the laboratories, wards, dispensary, amphitheatre and private operating rooms.

1. PATHOLOGY AND BACTERIOLOGY.

PATHOLOGY.

The instruction in Pathology is under the charge of Dr. W. H. Welch, Professor of Pathology, Johns Hopkins University, and of Dr. W. T. Councilman, Associate in Pathology and Associate Professor of Anatomy, Johns Hopkins University. It is conducted in the Pathological Laboratory, which is one of the buildings of the Johns Hopkins Hospital, especially constructed for pathological work. Here are to be found an autopsy theatre, rooms for bacteriological and special research, rooms for pathological histology, experimental pathology and photography and a museum.

Courses of instruction in Pathological Histology are continued throughout the academic year. In connection with the course in Pathological Histology fresh pathological specimens are demonstrated and also studied microscopically, especially by the aid of frozen sections. Instruction is also given in the methods of making post-mortem examinations and of recording the same.

Much attention is given to the collection and study of material in Comparative Pathology.

The resources of the laboratory are open to those who are fitted to engage in special investigations in any department of pathology.

In addition to regular practical courses in the laboratory extending throughout the academic year, special courses of lectures on pathological subjects will be given during the months of January and February, 1890 Professor Welch at this time will lecture once a week upon the Pathology of Diseases of the Heart and Blood Vessels. The subjects of fatty heart, fibrous myocarditis, diseases of the coronary arteries of the heart, thrombosis, embolism, infarction, and endarteritis, will be considered.

Professor Councilman will lecture upon Inflammation. The modern doctrines of inflammation, the origin of pus, the behavior of fixed cells in inflammation, the relation of bacteria to inflammation, are among the subjects to be considered. The lectures will be illustrated by gross and microscopical specimens.

BACTERIOLOGY.

The instruction in Bacteriology is under the charge of Professor W. H. Welch and of Dr. A. C. Abbott, Assistant in Bacteriology and Hygiene.

The rooms for bacteriological work are in the Pathological Laboratory. They are supplied with all of the apparatus required by modern bacteriological methods, such as those employed in the Hygienic Institute in Berlin. The laboratory has a full set of cultures of pathogenic micro-organisms, and of others useful for study and teaching.

Opportunities for studying bacteriology are available for students during the entire academic year, the laboratory being open on week days from nine o'clock in the morning until six in the evening. As much time can be given to the work as the student has at his disposal.

In the bacteriological course the student becomes familiar with the preparation of the various culture media, with the principles and methods of sterilization, and with the morphological and biological characters of the micro-organisms which belong to this

The start of medical education did not have to wait for the actual opening of the Johns Hopkins University School of Medicine. As seen from this notice in the first issue of The Johns Hopkins Hospital Bulletin, *instruction began with the opening of the hospital.*

There is a widespread hope and expectation that these combined institutions will endeavor to produce investigators as well as practitioners, to give to the world men who can not only sail by the old charts, but who can make new and better ones for the use of others. This can only be done where the professors and teachers are themselves seeking to increase knowledge, and doing this for the sake of the knowledge itself;—and hence it is supposed that from this Hospital will issue papers and reports giving accounts of advances in, and of new methods of acquiring knowledge, obtained in its wards and laboratories, and that thus all scientific men and all physicians shall share in the benefits of the work actually done within these walls.

—John Shaw Billings[3]

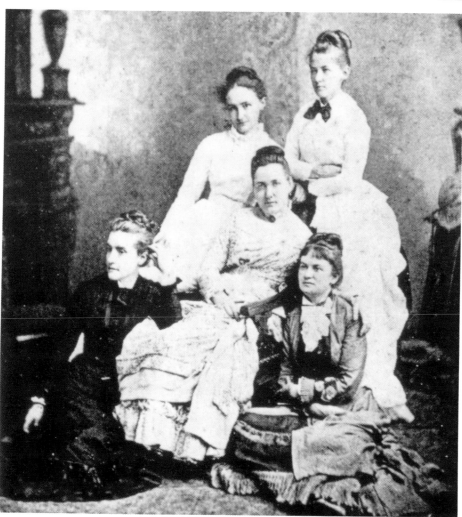

The medical school could not have opened without the money provided by Mary E. Garrett and the Women's Fund Committee. In a series of gifts, Garrett and this determined group of women, led by M. Carey Thomas, donated the necessary funds. Their money came with two stipulations: that admission be restricted to well-trained applicants with a bachelor's degree, and that women be admitted to the medical school on the same terms as men.

Four of the women who were most influential in raising the money were daughters of Hopkins trustees. Mary Garrett seated in the center, surrounded by (clockwise from lower left) Elizabeth King, Julia Rogers, Mary Gwinn, and M. Carey Thomas.

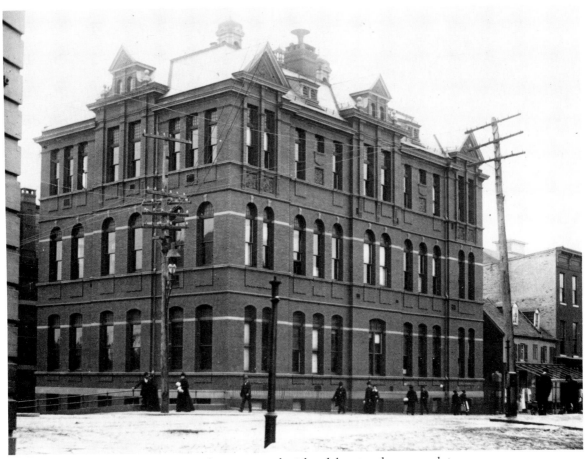

The medical school opened without an auditorium or a physiology laboratory large enough to accommodate all its students. The first class of medical students assembled to hear the dean's welcoming remarks in the Biological Laboratory on North Eutaw Street, on the original university campus. The Biological Laboratory was also used for instruction in physiology in these early years, but the students found the journey to and from the hospital an inconvenience. This situation persisted until 1898, when the facilities of the medical school were at last united on the East Baltimore campus.

When the Biological Laboratory opened in 1884, it was said to be the first such structure in this country devoted entirely to research and instruction in biology. Here, Henry Newell Martin, the first professor of biology in the university, welcomed the newly arrived William H. Welch and offered him temporary space until his Pathology Building was completed in 1886.

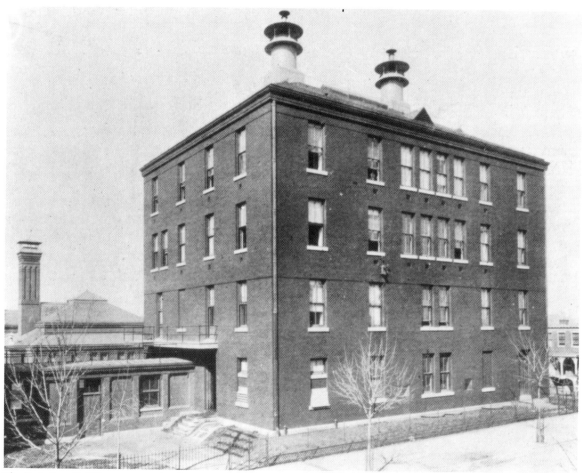

The Pathology Building contained only two stories when it was ready for use in 1886. Just before the medical school opened, two more stories were added to provide teaching space for anatomy and pharmacology. When the medical school opened in 1893, the Pathology Building housed all the preclinical sciences, with the exception of physiology. Franklin P. Mall occupied the fourth floor, and John J. Abel's pharmacology laboratory was located on the third.

The change from darker to lighter bricks reveals the addition of the third and fourth floors. The small white flag hanging from the window in the photograph at right was the signal to medical students and physicians that an autopsy was in progress.

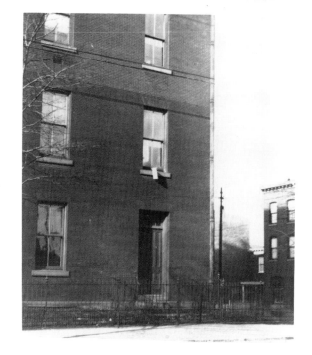

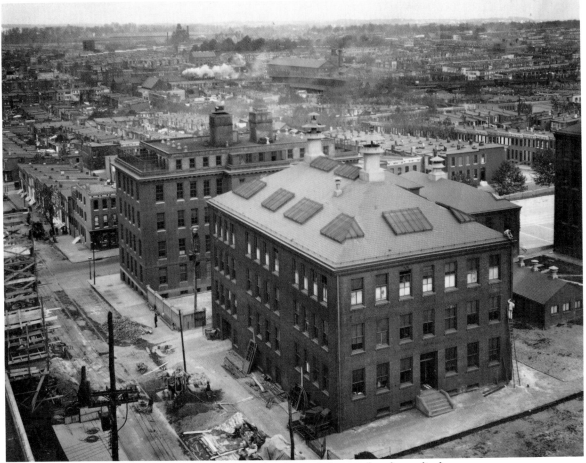

The faculty of the preclinical departments felt confined and crowded soon after the medical school opened. In 1897, the Department of Anatomy moved into the Women's Fund Memorial Building (known more informally as the anatomy building), which was constructed especially for the department's use.

Located on the medical school lot near the corner of Monument and Wolfe streets, the building comprised three stories, an attic, and a basement. Franklin P. Mall, the professor of anatomy, was determined to have adequate facilities for both dissection and the study of histology. He therefore planned a series of small rooms for dissection, but he shunned lectures almost completely. The building nevertheless contained a lecture hall large enough to accommodate the entire first-year class; it was used by other members of the department.

The zoologists and botanists have long ago learned the absurdity of the lecture method of teaching, but the anatomist patiently keeps up this slow and stupid method of instruction. It is stupid because no anatomist would use this same method if he were to learn instead of to teach.
—Franklin P. Mall[4]

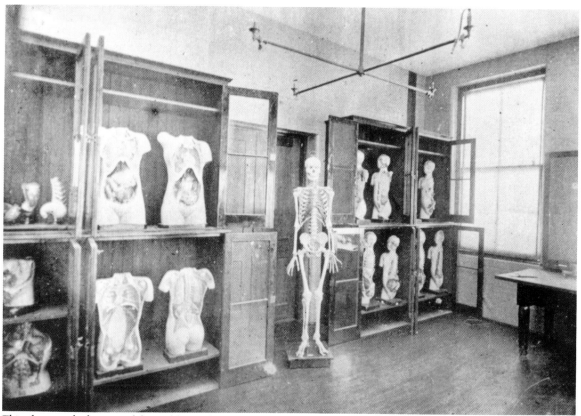

This photograph shows models used by students in the dissecting rooms of the third floor.

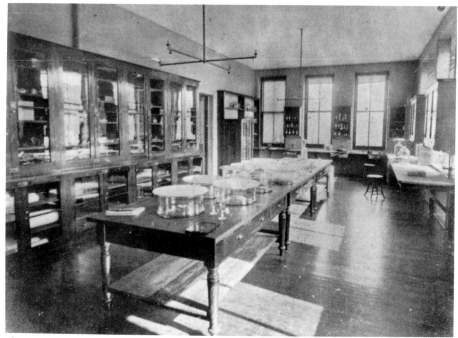

This spacious private laboratory on the second floor of the Women's Fund Memorial Building shows the extent to which the school supported the faculty's research.

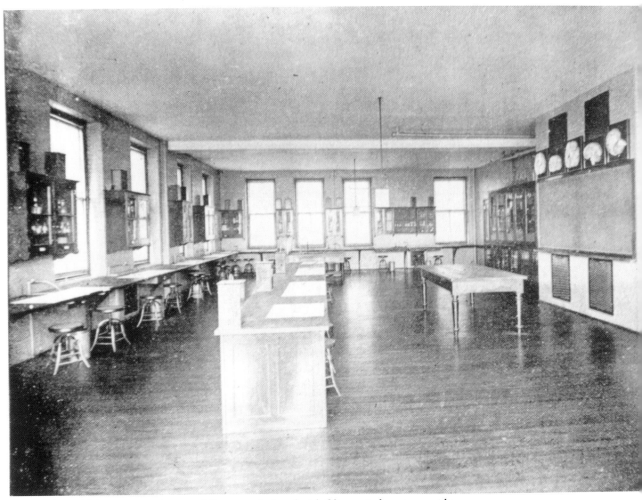

The histological laboratory on the second floor was designed with fifteen windows to provide light for thirty students.

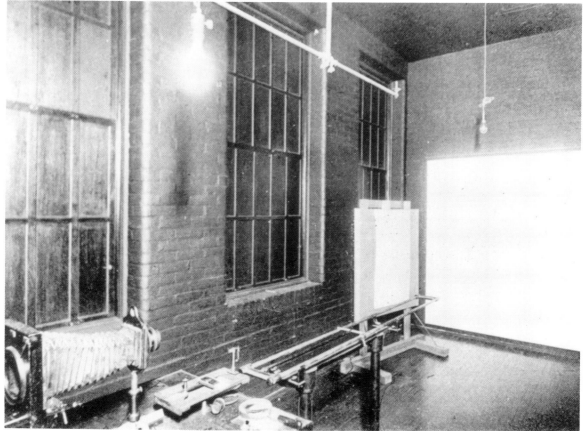

Medical photography became increasingly important in the years after the opening of the school of medicine, as this scene of the projection room in the anatomy department shows. This room on the ground floor contains elaborate equipment for holding specimens and for projecting their images on a screen.

A pioneer of medical photography was A. S. Murray, who worked mainly in the operating rooms in the early days of the Johns Hopkins Hospital.

In surgical cases intended for publication the photograph is an invaluable adjunct, either as a direct reproduction, or as an accurate basis for a careful drawing, which will in this way preserve the life and individuality of the subject, often lost in drawings hurriedly made and later finished from memory.

A further and possibly a still more important field for photography in gynecology is one which has been for the first time brought into use in the Johns Hopkins Hospital—that is, an effort by this means to crystallize a sufficient number of important steps during an operation from commencement to completion, so that by producing the photographs in the same order, a fairly accurate conception of the operator's methods may be obtained, and in this way the pictures will afford a basis for a vivid lecture.

—A. S. Murray[5]

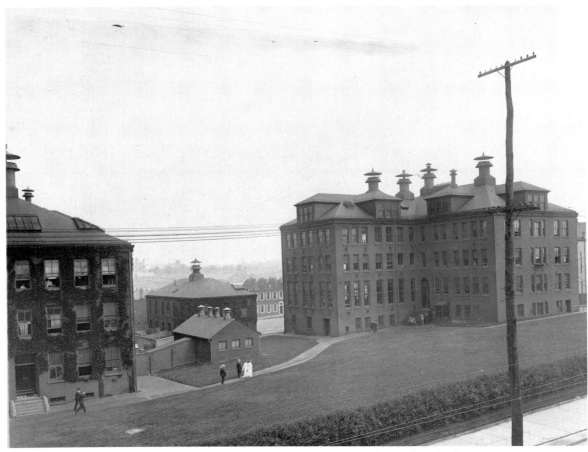

With the inclusion of three major subjects in the first-year curriculum, crowding at the school of medicine became acute. In 1897, construction was started on a building that would house the departments of Physiology, Pharmacology, and Physiological Chemistry. The Physiology Building (later known as the "Old Physiology Building") was located on the east end of the medical school property. It followed the architectural pattern of the Women's Fund Memorial Building; both buildings were constructed of brick and lacked any architectural adornment.

The new building opened in 1898. On its first floor were offices for the dean and registrar, an expanded library for the medical school, and an auditorium, which was later used as the principal teaching laboratory of the physiology department. The Department of Physiology was located on the second floor and the Department of Pharmacology on the third. Instruction in physiological chemistry (which was not yet a separate department) was carried out in student laboratories on the third floor, and later in the attic.

This view of the medical school side of the campus, ca. 1912, shows the Women's Fund Memorial Building at the left, the smaller Hunterian Laboratory (built in 1905) in the middle, and the Physiology Building on the right.

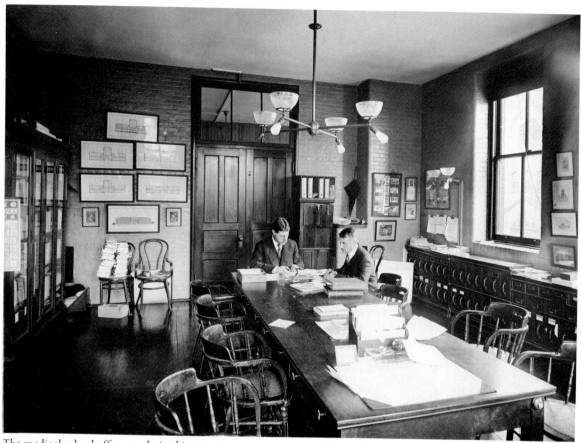

The medical school offices early in this century were a simple affair in comparison with those of later decades. J. Whitridge Williams and George J. Coy, the long-time registrar of the medical school, comprised the "administration" between 1911 and 1922. They are shown here in the dean's office.

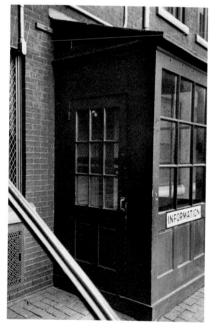

Students visiting the office of the dean used this modest entrance to the Physiology Building for several decades.

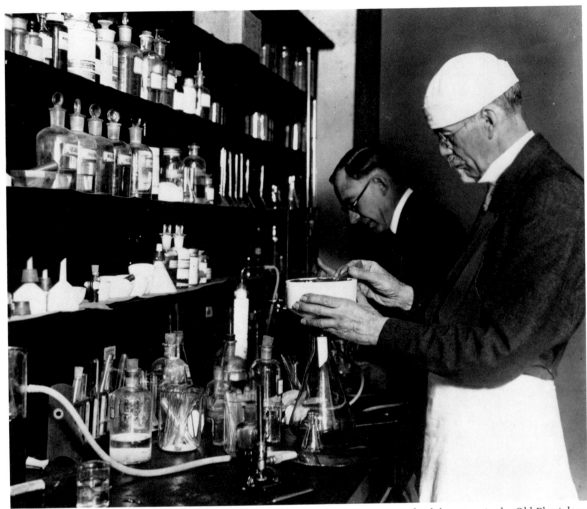

John J. Abel, the first professor of pharmacology, appears in his laboratory in the Old Physiology Building, ca. 1915. The accompanying sketch shows an experimental artificial kidney designed and built by Abel and first used on animals in his laboratory in 1913. In its earliest form, the vividiffusion apparatus, as he called it, contained sixteen tubes. The arterial cannula is marked with an arrow leading into the apparatus; the venous cannula arises from the tube with the arrow pointing outward.

Abel's vividiffusion experiments were carried out in dogs, one of which is shown on the lawn of the Hunterian Laboratory. It was not until several decades later that this technique was used in the treatment of renal failure in man.

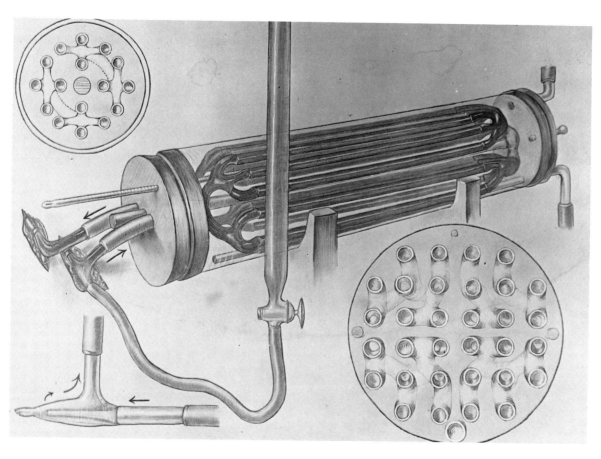

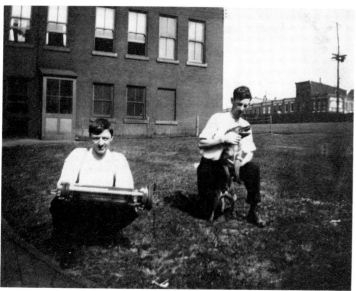

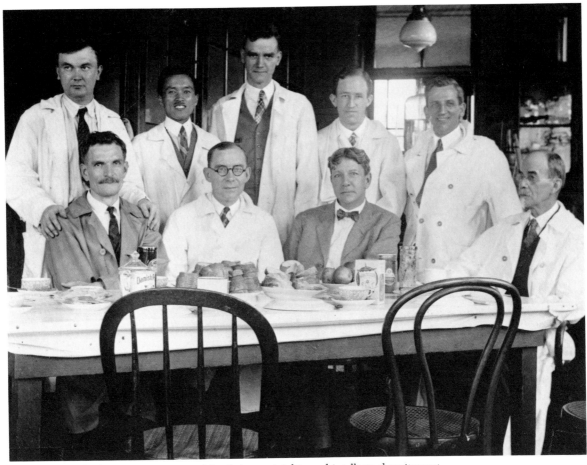

Lunches in Abel's department were noted for their conviviality and intellectual excitement. A scene at Abel's famous lunch table is shown here: (left to right, seated) C. A. Rouiller, E. M. K. Geiling, W. W. Ford, John J. Abel; (standing) J. V. Supniewski, T. Ishikawa, Frederick Bell, Vincent Vermooten, Sir David Campbell.

What astonished and immensely impressed me as a European during these first days after my arrival in the fall of 1926 was the friendly informality with which the professor treated the young research people and the technicians, and the free and relaxed atmosphere pervading the whole place, which contrasted so strongly with that engendered by the rank-conscious, hierarchic system under which I was apprenticed. Indeed, my first encounter with "the Professor" made clear to me that things were different here in this respect. When I made my way up the stairs to the third floor I met him coming down, but I had,

of course, no inkling that the old gentleman with the white cap who looked like something of a cross between Uncle Sam and a Chinese Mandarin was the famous Professor Abel with whom I was to work. He gave me a friendly smile and what to me looked like a wink, which puzzled me a bit at the moment. He showed me into his office, put his arm around me, and said, "I am so glad, my boy, that you have come; we have been looking forward to you." Certainly no Geheimrat or Hofrat would ever have given a young nobody a reception like that, and it made a deep and lasting impression on me.

—E. M. K. Geiling[6]

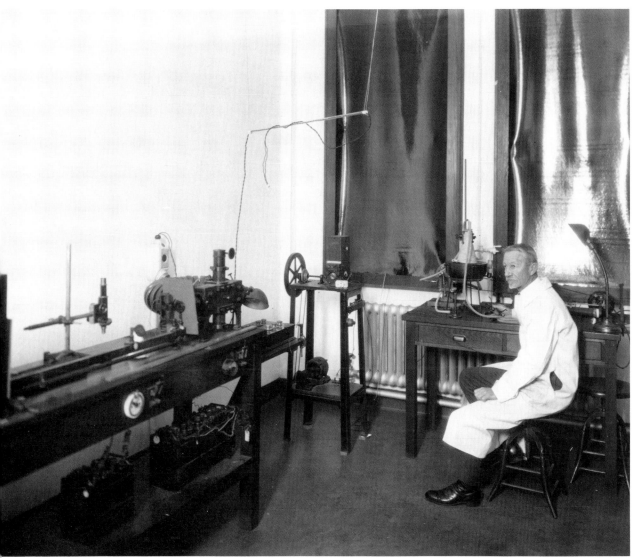

William Henry Howell, America's pioneer in blood coagulation studies and the first professor of physiology at the medical school, is shown in his laboratory.

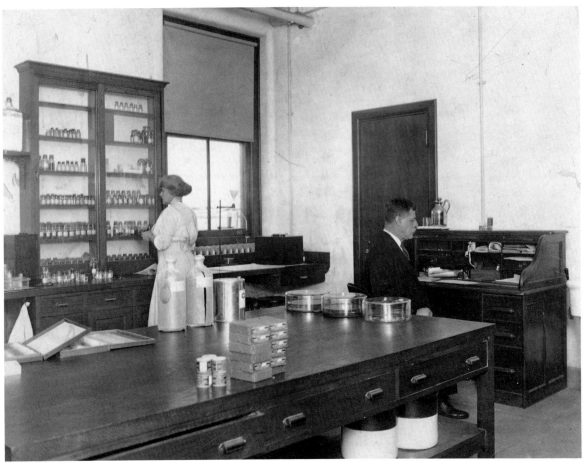

J. Whitridge Williams served simultaneously as dean of the medical school and professor of obstetrics at Hopkins. He is shown here with Mrs. Williams in his laboratory.

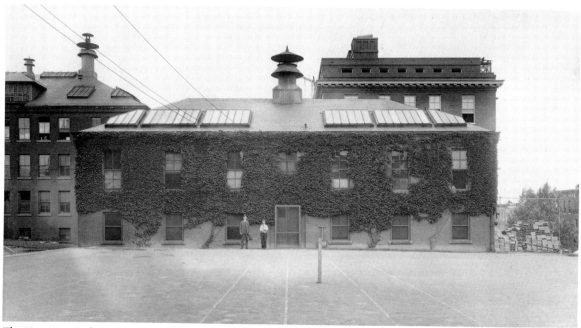

The Hunterian Laboratory, or "Old Hunterian," as it came to be known, was a rectangular, two-story brick structure on the medical school lot between the Anatomy and Physiology buildings. It had its own paddock for animals; a well-lighted room for student operating teams, research rooms for faculty of the departments of Surgery, Pathology, and Medicine, and the usual supporting quarters for research, including animal rooms.

The teaching exercises and research activities in these laboratories were a hallmark of the early years of medicine at Johns Hopkins. As Franklin P. Mall wrote in reference to his Department of Anatomy, "The object of the laboratory is to teach students, to train investigators, and to investigate." This was the guiding philosophy of the medical school as a whole, and nowhere was it better illustrated than in the rooms of the Hunterian Laboratory.

The Hunterian had been built at the behest of Harvey Cushing, of the Department of Surgery, and William G. MacCallum, a member of the Department of Pathology. The name "Hunterian" paid homage to John Hunter, the British experimental surgeon of the eighteenth century.

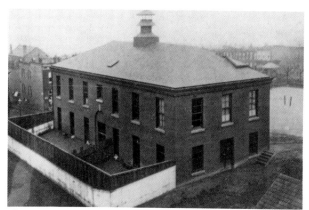

These views of the Hunterian Laboratory reveal the east front of the building and the paddock at the rear. Note the extensive use of skylights, whose effects are more evident in the interior scenes.

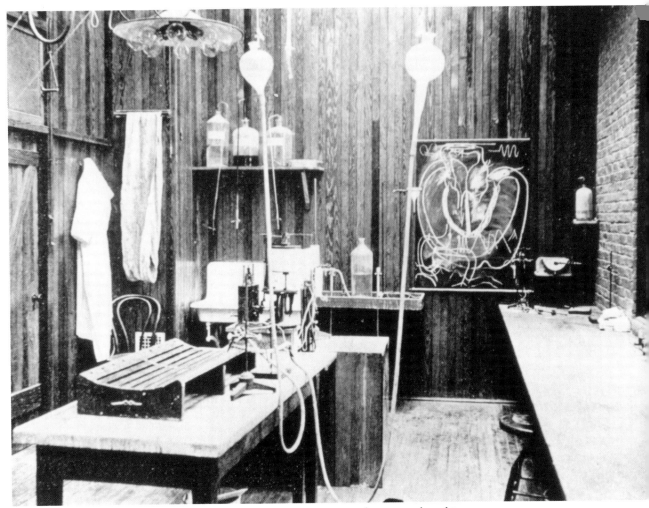

Cushing and MacCallum used the facilities of the Hunterian to accommodate research and instruction in surgery and in pathology. This laboratory, assigned to pathology, was the site of the experiments of MacCallum and Carl Voegtlin on the relation of calcium to the parathyroid gland, and of MacCallum's investigation of the role of the islets of Langerhans in carbohydrate metabolism.

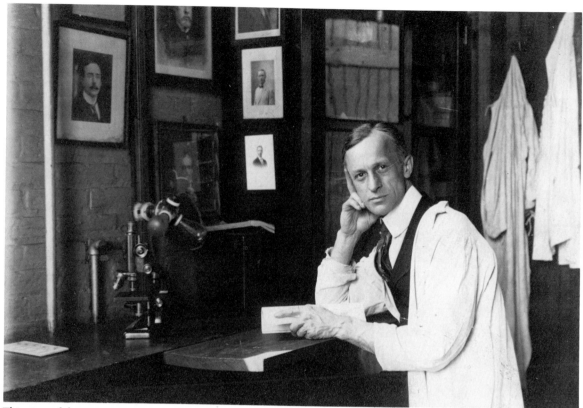

This view of the pensive Harvey Cushing shows him at this desk in the Hunterian in 1907.

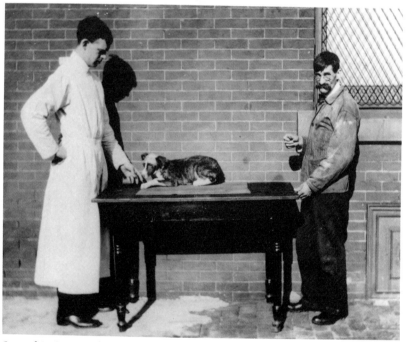

Samuel J. Crowe, who assisted Harvey Cushing with his experimental work on the pituitary gland, is shown with "Jimmy the Diener" and a hypophysectomized dog in 1910.

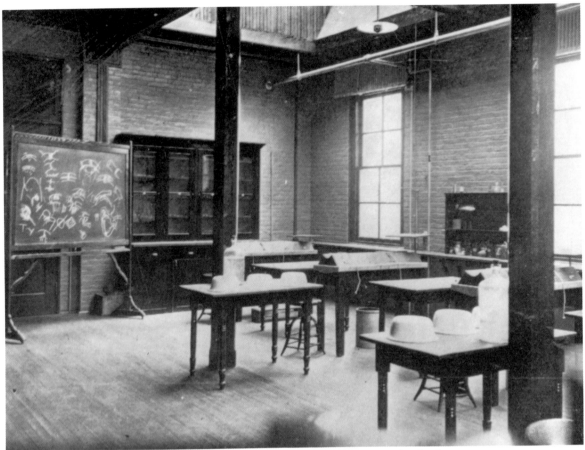

In the Hunterian Laboratory, Harvey Cushing initiated his course in dog surgery for third-year medical students. Halsted had devised the course, but he had turned it over to Cushing shortly after Cushing's return to Baltimore in the fall of 1901. For several years, it was taught in the room that became Florence Sabin's laboratory in the Department of Anatomy, but in 1905 the course was moved to the Hunterian.

It was then, with a view of teaching our students of Medicine the first principles of operative technique, of which the all-important element is asepsis—for a surgeon's most active reflex must react to uncleanliness—at the same time that they were learning as much as possible of the diseases which in themselves or through their complications are supposedly amenable to operative measures, that this operative course was first inaugurated.

—Harvey Cushing[7]

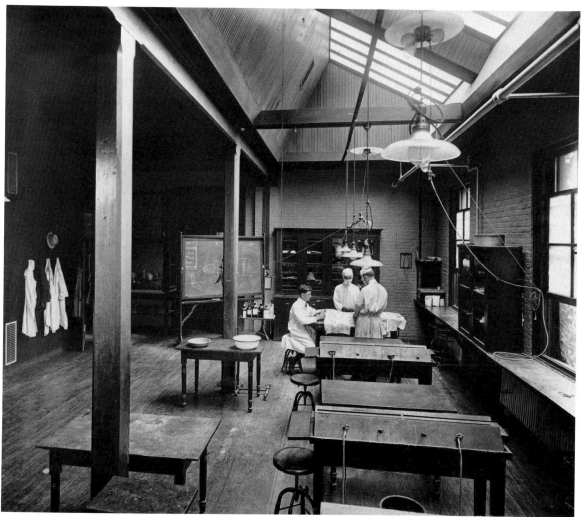

Cushing believed that the key principles of surgery—which included diagnosis, proper sterile technique, handling the tissues in careful dissection, and proper control of bleeding vessels— could all be learned only on the living animal. Surgical anatomy and technique might be learned on the cadaver, but a living operative subject was required to give the students a proper appreciation of the complexities of surgery and its effects on the tissues of the living body.

But when we come to treatment, it is a different matter. A student may read surgery, may hear and see surgery; and yet, without having himself practiced operations and those on the living body, he remains totally incapable of carrying out those measures which alone distinguish this branch of medicine. One would not expect to play the violin after a course of lectures on music and merely by watching a performer for a few semesters. . . .

These twenty men are divided into units of five, and each of these units comprises a non-operating physician, an operator, his first and second assistant and an anaesthetist. At each succeeding exercise the members rotate in these positions; the "family physician," for example, becoming the surgeon, the surgeon the first assistant, and so on. . . .

I am far from claiming that this method will make more surgeons out of a body of students, but it will, I believe, make the future physician more appreciative of the surgical point of view; more capable of understanding when handicraft

may with propriety be called for, and the only safe methods of applying it; able, too, in case of need, to put his own hands to the work. . . .

They learn, at the same time, to keep records; to present and discuss case histories intelligently; to visualize from such a history the actual condition of the patient. They learn to prepare all of the supplies necessary for an operation and by actual experience the way of conducting it. They learn to appreciate the risks of anaesthesia, and the need of untiring concentration upon his task by the administrator thereof. They learn to care kindly and properly for a living patient, in whose uneventful recovery as great personal pride will be taken as chagrin will be felt in case of complications for which some unavoidable error or neglect may have been responsible. They learn to describe their own operative procedures, to look up the literature of the subject, and are supplied with a stimulus for investigating experimentally the causes of such conditions as may still have an obscure etiology.

—Harvey Cushing[8]

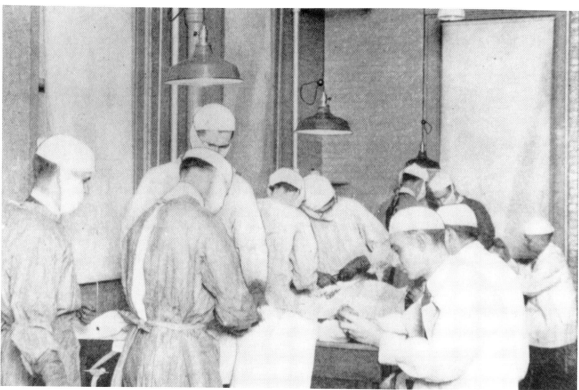

Interior scene from the operating room of the Hunterian. All but the anesthetist are in gowns, caps, masks, and gloves. This building had excellent natural illumination as well as electric light.

By our collegiate degrees we are—in this country at least—all Doctors of Medicine, and should a surgeon's hands become maimed he surely could continue the practice of medicine. On the other hand, it is highly essential for the one who is disinclined to operate "in large doses" to have just as thorough an understanding of the limitations and possibilities of major surgical procedures as the operator himself possesses, for a knowledge of surgery does not necessarily entail its practice. . . .

How can the "born physician" be brought to better appreciate and have the more patience with operative measures? How can the natural craftsman, on the other hand, be made to realize that he is likewise a physician and be led to moderate his activities within bounds, so that he may become more worthy of the position that his successes have forced from the medical faculties of earlier times? These results, I think, may in a

measure be brought about by a different method of presenting the subject to the student; by making him realize that surgery is only a form of therapy—a form of therapy entailing great responsibilities and therefore not a thing to be made a show of before a crowded amphitheatre—and that the operator's duties and his relations to medicine and to his patient are the same as those of the "physician," with whom he must share alike an understanding of the general pathology of disease, and the recognition of its symptoms; that he owes it to his profession not to make his chosen branch of it a trade; and furthermore by urging upon those, who by nature are not particularly fitted for and have no learning whatsoever toward manipulative practices in medicine, their even greater need of acquiring, during their student days, as much familiarity as possible with this branch of the healing art.

—Harvey Cushing[9]

. . . Dr. Welch described Sargent as grouping his four sitters, over and over again, before he was satisfied. Sometimes he requested two of the doctors to stand, and then only one of them. He changed their positions, again and again. Before he began to paint, however, he settled upon the grouping that is shown in the completed portrait, and this, as Dr. Welch said, disposes of the assertion made by some critics that the composition had taken its form by accident and as the work proceeded. Dr. Welch also noted that the enlargement of the canvas by a piece joined at the side and another at the top was not unforeseen, but was mentioned by Sargent at the outset as a thing he expected to have done. The grouping, then, and the scale of the portrait were fixed by the artist when he began and so the sitters went on to do their part. They were sometimes all together in the studio, but not often. Sometimes three of them sat, sometimes two of them, but more often each doctor was posed by himself. Dr. Welch's head was painted practically in one sitting. He was struck by Sargent's unobtrusive way of studying him; he never felt that he was being closely scrutinized. Sargent talked constantly while he was at work, smoked innumerable cigarettes, and was always walking to and fro. When Dr. Welch asked him about his exercise, he said laughingly that he had once estimated that he walked about four miles a day in his studio. Though Dr. Welch's head was painted so quickly, the painter was not equally swift in his treatment of all the other sitters. Dr. Osler, especially, had to give sitting after sitting.

The work went forward, on the whole, with great smoothness. There were some difficulties, as when the portrait of Dr. Osler struck them all as a failure and Sargent painted it out and did it all over again. But then everything seemed to move swimmingly. Just at this time Sargent himself suddenly grew discouraged. He paused one day, and knitting his brow, and lifting his hand with a gesture of bewilderment, he said, "It won't do. It isn't a picture. I cannot see just what to do, but it isn't a picture." He stood for a little while thinking it over, and presently the clouds seemed to pass. He asked if there would be anything incongruous about the introduction of a large, old Venetian globe into the background. It was in his other studio, he said, and he would have it brought around if it were permissible. Of course it was; and a day or two after, the globe was there. It was so large that he had to have the doorway chopped to let it into the room. (That was very like Sargent; he would have had an entire wall removed if it had been necessary in making the portrait a perfect work of art.) When they sat again with the globe in the background, Sargent studied the group with anxious interest, and then, in a swift stroke, drew the silhouette of the thing on the canvas. "We have got our picture," he said, and the portrait as it stands shows with that unerring instinct he had thought of the one thing fitted to serve his purpose.

Dr. Welch had some very interesting things to say about the color scheme. He asked Sargent if he could wear his Yale robe, and the painter immediately acquiesced; but when Dr. Osler spoke of wearing his red Oxford robe, Sargent humorously forbade it, saying:

"No, I can't paint you in that. It won't do. I know all about that red. You know they gave me a degree down there, and I've got one of those robes." Musingly, he went on. "I've left it on the roof in the rain. I've buried it in the garden. It's no use. The red is as red as ever. The stuff is too good. It won't fade. Now, if you could get a Dublin degree? The red robes there are made of different stuff and if you wash them they come down to a beautiful pink. Do you think you could get a Dublin degree?—No, I couldn't paint you in that Oxford red! Why, do you know they say that the women who work on the red coats worn by the British soldiers have all sorts of trouble with their eyes, etc., etc."

—Royal Cortissoz[10]

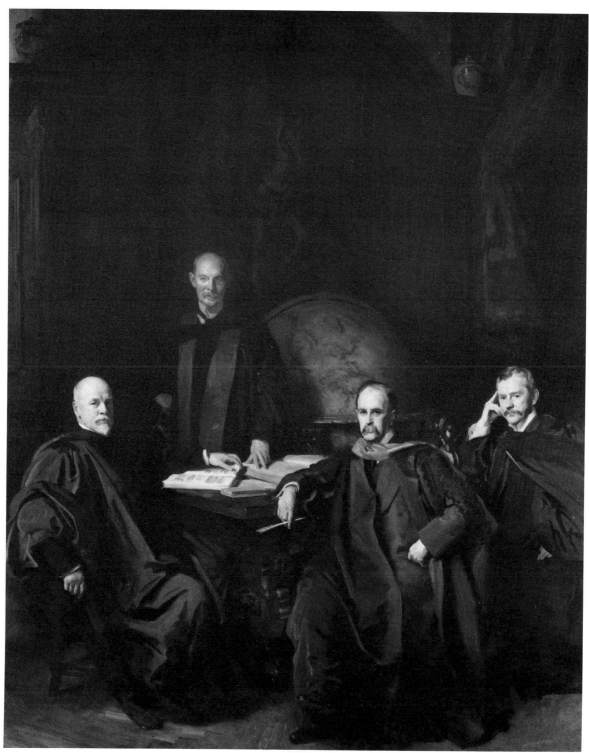

This famous portrait of the original clinical faculty was painted by John Singer Sargent in 1906. The painting was commissioned by Mary E. Garrett and presented to the University in 1907. It now hangs in the William H. Welch Medical Library. The portrait shows (left to right) Welch, William Halsted, William Osler, and Howard Kelly.

3

THE HOSPITAL'S FIRST
TWENTY-FIVE YEARS, 1889–1914

Section 3 follows the Johns Hopkins Hospital from its founding to 1914, the year of its twenty-fifth anniversary. By then, most of the innovations that characterized medicine at Johns Hopkins were in place.

The success of the hospital in attracting patients and staff soon overburdened its original facilities, and new buildings were constructed to accommodate the large number of patients. When the hospital opened in 1889, it had 250 beds. At the end of its first quarter of a century, the hospital had inpatient accommodations for 625.[1]

Just before the opening of the school of medicine in 1893, two additional hospital wards, M and O, were constructed for black patients. Before the construction of these two separate wards, black patients had occupied one cordoned-off section in each of the five public wards.

As for the outpatients, by 1914, more than 300 patients a day were being seen in the outpatient clinic, a number that made Winford Smith, the hospital's director, approach the Trustees with a request for a larger dispensary.

But what makes an institution great, Daniel C. Gilman wrote, was "men, not buildings," and at the twenty-fifth anniversary celebration, Judge Henry D. Harlan, the president of the Board of Trustees, reemphasized Gilman's motto:

Large as is the property under our care (though it is inadequate to enable us to advance into fields of usefulness that are constantly opening), the greatest endowment which the Hospital has is the spirit of loyalty and service that pervades its staff and its employees. It is their devotion, their zeal, their cooperation, their skill, their learning and their ability which have brought it into prominence and made it useful.[2]

As William Osler pointed out on the same occasion, twenty-five years is hardly even a generation. Yet in that span of time, the principles described in the companion volume were firmly established in the hospital and school of medicine and became a model for others to emulate. Osler summarized the importance of this first quarter of a century:

The feeling, however, is strong, too strong to be passed over, that the year 1889 did mean something in the history of medicine in this country. One thing certainly it meant, as originally designed by that great leader Daniel C. Gilman, that the ideals of the men on this side of the Jones Falls were to be the same as those of the men in the laboratories of North Howard Street, that a type of medical school was to be created new to this country, in which teacher and student alike should be in the fighting line. That is lesson number one of our first quarter century, judged by which we stand or fall. And lesson number two was the demonstration that the student of medicine has his place in the hospital as part of its machinery just as much as he has in the anatomical laboratory, and that to combine successfully in his education practice with science, the academic freedom of the university must be transplanted to the hospital.[3]

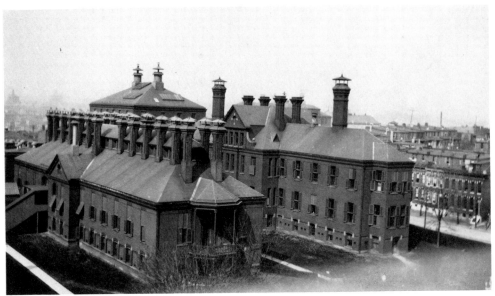

By 1896, the need for inpatient maternity facilities had become pressing. To create a lying-in ward, the southern end of the Isolating Ward was bricked off by a solid wall. This photograph shows both the Maternity Ward and Wards M and O, which appear at the right of the photograph. The Isolating Ward maintained an entrance (left) separate from the entrance to the lying-in ward.

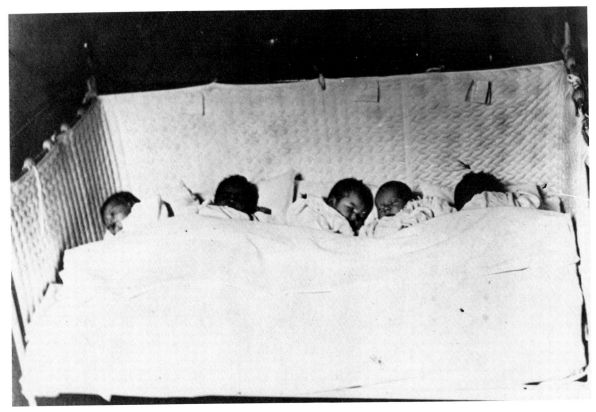

This photograph of infants in the nursery dates from 1903.

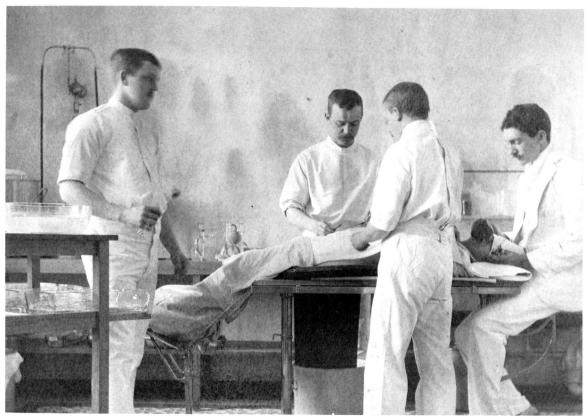

When the hospital opened in 1889, the Gynecological Operating Room was at the center of the second floor of Ward B, which was later remodeled to house the Wilmer Institute of Ophthalmology.

The personal operating table of Howard A. Kelly, gynecologist-in-chief, had a brass frame with a thick glass top. Kelly appears at the center of the photograph, performing a laparotomy. His second assistant is at the far left. Hunter Robb, Kelly's chief assistant, is second from the right, and William W. Russell, the anesthetist, is at the far right of the photograph. Note that the surgeons are not wearing rubber gloves or masks.

Less than three years after the opening of the hospital, Kelly already needed larger facilities. Because of the rapid increase in the number of gynecological procedures Kelly was performing, the Trustees decided in 1891 to erect a building to be used exclusively for gynecological surgery. This building was the first addition to the original hospital plans. It occupied the site intended for a bath house, one of the planned structures in the southern row of pavilions.

Construction required only one year, and the new building was finished in 1892. Later, when the original private ward for women was converted to the Wilmer Ophthalmological Institute, the erstwhile Gynecological Operating Room was joined to it by an entrance lobby connected to the Wilmer's main corridor.

Show me a man's operating room, and I will tell you of the character of his work.
—Howard A. Kelly[4]

The new Gynecological Operating Room was built to Kelly's specifications. He had listed four essentials:[5]

It should be well-lighted.
It should be easy to clean thoroughly.
It should have an unlimited supply of hot and cold water.
Instruments and other necessities should be within easy reach.

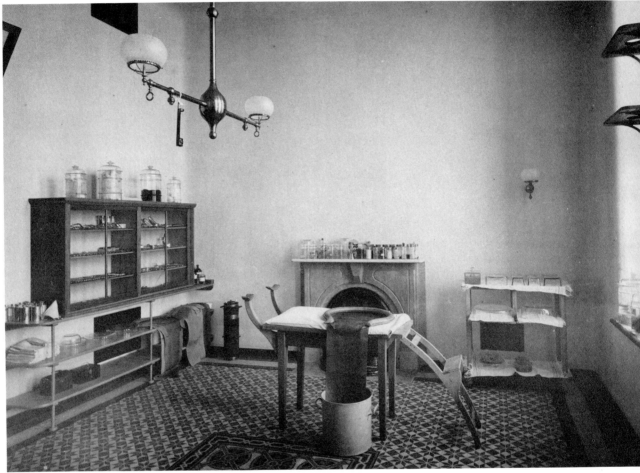

The south end of the gynecological operating room, with the laparotomy table with ovariotomy pad in place, an instrument case on the left, and a moveable carriage for instruments on the right.

I do not believe the history of medicine presents a parallel to the munificence of our colleague Kelly to his clinic. Equal in bulk, in quality, and in far-reaching practical value to the work from any department of the University, small wonder that his clinic became the Mecca for surgeons from all parts of the world, that his laboratory methods, perfected by Drs. Cullen and Hurdon, have become general models. . . .

—William Osler[6]

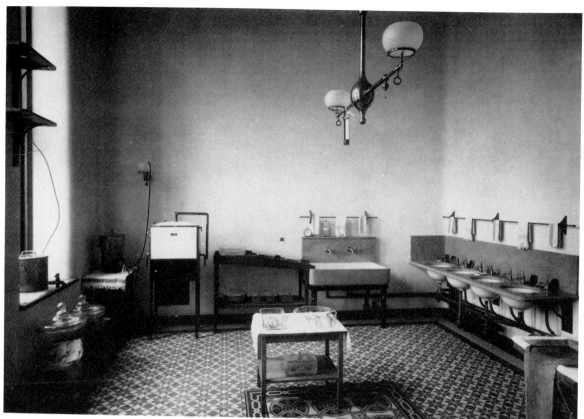

The other end of the operating room. Left to right: jars for bandages and towels, a steam sterilizer, and porcelain sinks for washing instruments.

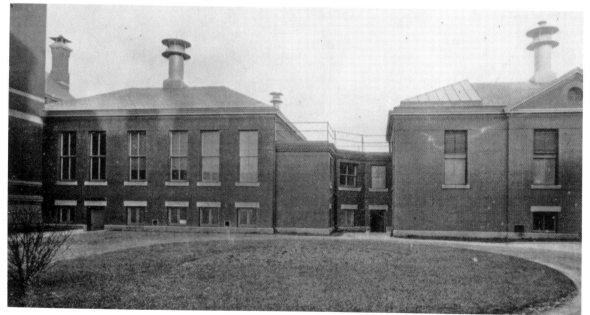

An addition to this gynecological operating room was completed in 1897 with funds provided by Kelly. In these enlarged quarters, the Department of Gynecology carried on its surgical work until completion of the new Woman's Clinic in 1927.

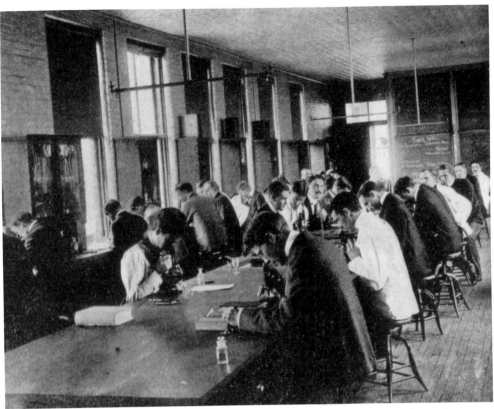

The plans for the Johns Hopkins Hospital were marred by one striking omission: the hospital planners forgot to include space for clinical laboratories. As a result, two temporary laboratories—one for routine tests and one for student teaching and investigation—were set up in the basement.

These laboratories were at the heart of Osler's plans for instruction in the Department of Medicine.

In 1896, when two classes had advanced to the clinical years, a new laboratory was built between the Amphitheater and the Dispensary on Monument Street. This 1901 photograph of a class in clinical microscopy was used by Osler in his classic article cited here.

A necessary adjunct to a modern hospital is the clinical laboratory, in which students can work, and in which they study systematically the methods of investigation of the blood, sputa, urine and secretions. Twice a week from two to four in the afternoon, the third-year class is drilled in these methods by Dr. Emerson, the resident physician in charge of the clinical laboratory. Familiarized thoroughly with the use of the microscope by prolonged laboratory courses in histology and pathology in the previous years, the student is ready to appreciate the modern clinical methods for investigating disease which are so essential in diagnosis. . . . I may remark that the clinical laboratory is in immediate proximity to the wards, and has accommodation for about 110 students. As each student has his own place throughout the session and his own microscope, the laboratory becomes in reality what its name indicates, and to it the student goes at his leisure to work at his specimens, or for private research. Conducted properly, with a protracted course and ample material, this class becomes one of the most popular, as it certainly is one of the most useful, in the curriculum.

—William Osler[7]

Student nurses, as well as medical students, took classes in the medical school buildings. Classroom instruction was a special feature of the school of nursing, which offered a rigorous academic program along with practical training.

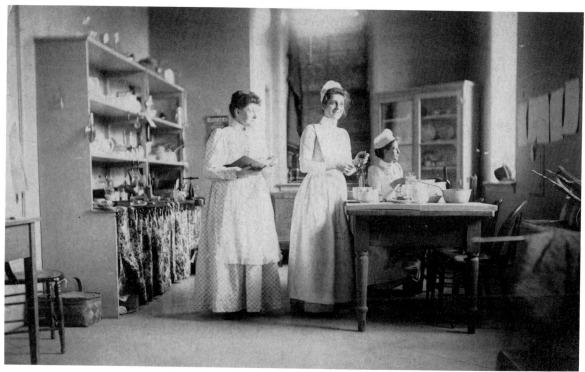

This photograph, taken ca. 1890, shows a class in nutrition for nursing students. In the center is Susan Mead, a nursing student who later married William S. Thayer of the Department of Medicine. At the left is Mary Boland, an instructor in the Boston Cooking School; seated is Georgia Nevins.

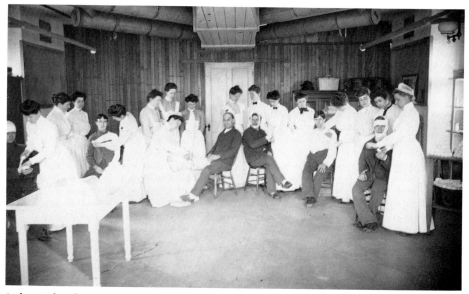

A class in bandaging.

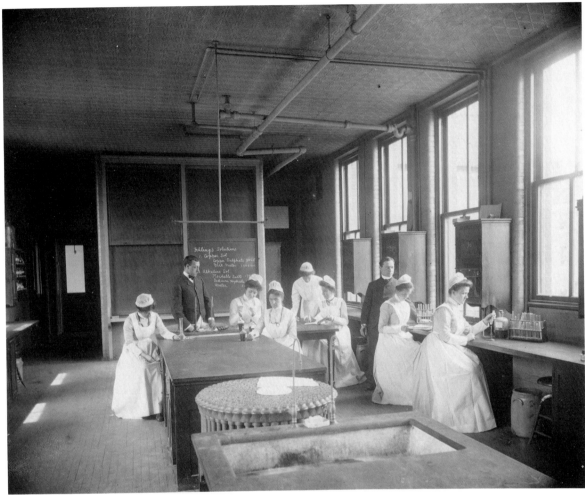

A class for nursing students in the clinical laboratory.

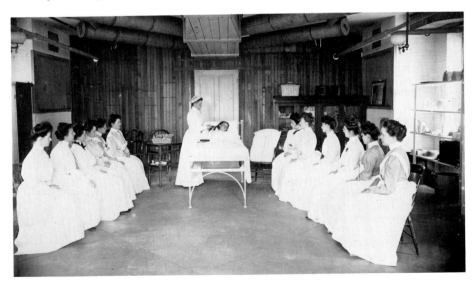

A class in bedside nursing.

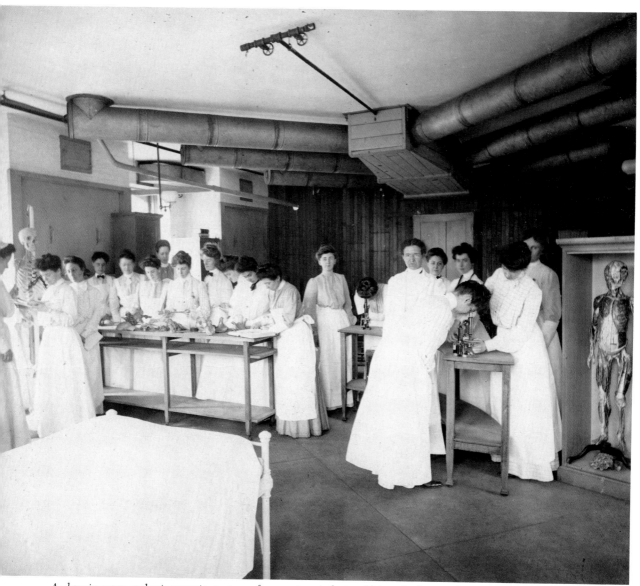

A class in gross and microscopic anatomy for nursing students which took place in the Women's Fund Memorial Building, ca. 1915. It was taught by Florence Sabin, who was the first woman to reach the rank of full professor in the medical school. Dr. Sabin, or "Flossie," as she was known to many classes of medical and nursing students, is at the right rear of the photograph, wearing glasses.

Like Howard A. Kelly's Gynecological Service, William S. Halsted's Department of Surgery flourished during the hospital's early years. Within a decade of the hospital's opening, Halsted's surgical service was already receiving worldwide recognition as a leading clinical school. Here Halsted and his residents devised new approaches to the cure of hernia and to the surgical treatment of breast cancer. Their innovative surgical techniques included a new intestinal suture and the use of rubber gloves. As Halsted trained an impressive array of young men, these talents were spread across the country.

Surgery, like the other clinical services, soon needed larger clinical facilities that would be specifically adapted to its work. Halsted prevailed upon the trustees to provide his department with an entire building.

This new, four-story surgical building had ample room for both teaching and surgical care of patients. The amphitheater was located on the first floor. On the second floor were rooms for accident cases, x-ray facilities, and a clinical laboratory. (Lewellys F. Barker's full-time research divisions in the Department of Medicine were also located on the second floor.) Laboratory space and classrooms were located on the third floor, and on the fourth floor there were well-lit operating rooms and the support services they required.

The building was opened in October 1904, with much fanfare. In his speech for the occasion, Judge Henry D. Harlan, the president of the hospital Board of Trustees, expressed the hope that this new building would "mark a new era in the advance and work of the Hospital."

To commemorate the opening of his new building, Halsted gathered his senior team for a well publicized and photographed operation—widely known as the "all-star" performance.[8] Two views are shown here.

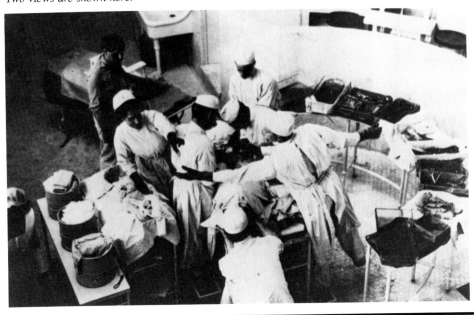

The staff which surrounds Dr. Halsted is composed of his senior assistants—it is not his regular resident staff. The Professor is operating on a patient with osteomyelitis of the upper end of the femur. I remember the case well. He was performing a resection. He is holding a wooden hammer bound with metal. Jim Mitchell was giving the anesthetic, I was the first assistant [directly across the table from Halsted with Cushing on Finney's right], Cushing, the second, Joe Bloodgood the third [on Halsted's right]. Hugh Young was the instrument man. Follis is disappearing in the background and F. H. Baetjer [Assistant Surgeon in charge of actinography] sits lost in contemplation on the steps. . . . The nurse is Miss Crawford. . . .

—J.M.T. Finney[9]

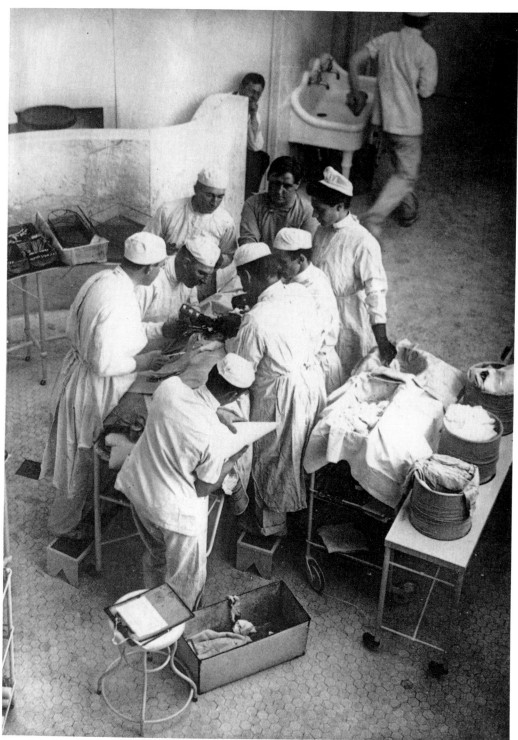

Note that the nurse, Miss Crawford, is gloved and assisting the surgeons directly. Before the 1890s, nurses were present to assist the patients, not the surgeons. As an increasing number of operations were performed, the role of nurses in the operating room changed, and they became responsible for passing instruments to the surgeon and "setting up the room" for the surgical procedure.[10]

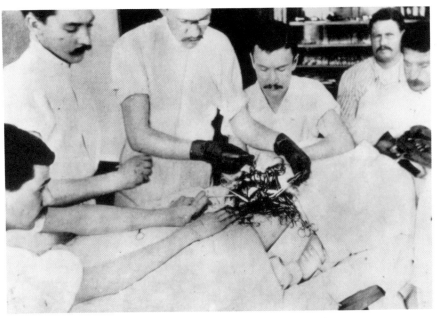

One of the earliest operations in which the surgeons used rubber gloves.

It was the custom on the surgical service to scrub the hands and arms vigorously with soap and water and then soak them for ten minutes in a basin filled with a 1:1000 mercuric chloride solution. This technique produced such a marked dermatitis on the hands of Miss Caroline Hampton, the head nurse in the surgical division (and later Mrs. Halsted) that in 1890 Dr. Halsted asked the Goodyear Rubber Company to make, as an experiment, two pairs of thin rubber gloves with gauntlets.

—Samuel J. Crowe[11]

Gloves in Halsted's operating room were in constant use by two members of the operative group and occasionally used by Halsted himself in operating upon joints, yet it was seven years (1896) before it became the practice of everyone who cleaned up for the operation to wear these gloves as a routine.

The moment this routine use of gloves was adopted the suppuration of closed wounds, for example in inguinal hernia, fell from more than 9 per cent to less than 0.5 per cent.

—Joseph Bloodgood[12]

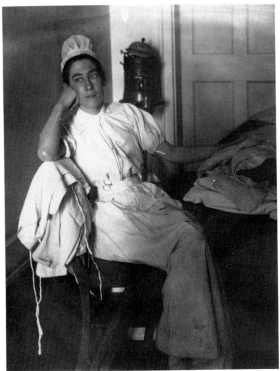

A surgical staff nurse ca. 1910. Note that gowns are ready for the surgeons, but the nurses are not yet wearing them.

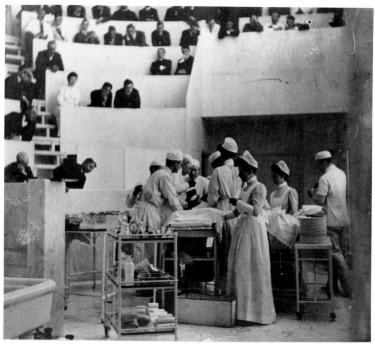

There had rarely been many onlookers in the old operating room, in the basement of Ward G, or even in the renovated operating room in an upper ward, which had the benefit of a large window. Here, the window directly faced the audience. The light reduced their pupils to pin-points, and they could see little more than shadows and Halsted's back. Similarly, the "all-star operation" was performed without an audience. But the main operating room in the new building had 180 seats, and onlookers became a regular feature at surgical procedures in the new building. They still faced the large windows that provided the main source of light, and some are evidently still straining to see.

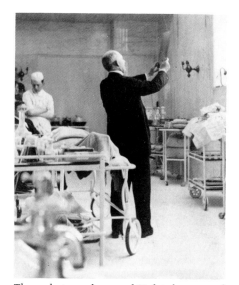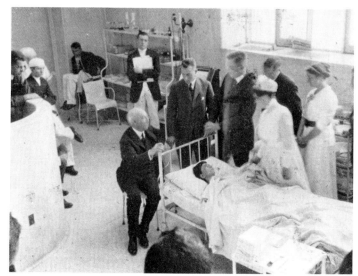

These photographs reveal Halsted as a teacher rather than in his usual surgical garb.

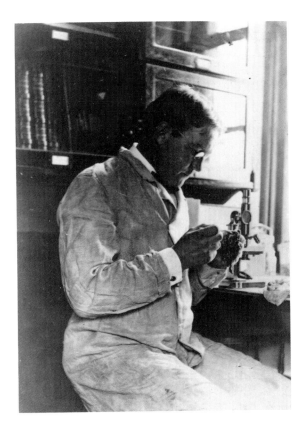

The research tradition was as strong in surgery as in any of the other clinical departments, and the new surgical building, as well as the Hunterian Laboratory, contained extensive facilities for scientific investigation.

This photograph of Joseph Bloodgood, one of Halsted's early residents, shows him in his laboratory in the new surgical building, in the late 1910s or early 1920s.

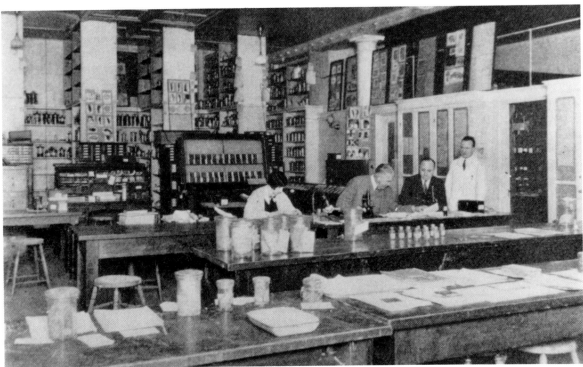

The large surgical pathology laboratory in the new surgical building remained in operation until the building was demolished to make way for the Blalock Building.

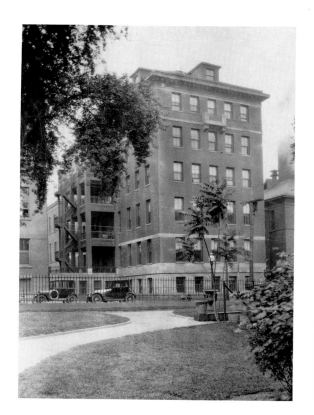

Urology began to develop as a separate part of surgery shortly after 1898, when Halsted appointed Hugh H. Young as urologist-in-chief. The clinic for urological cases was located in the basement of the new surgical building, opened in 1904.

One of Young's most grateful patients was the colorful New York bachelor businessman, James Buchanan Brady. Brady was fond of jewelry and lavish dress and has been known by his nickname, "Diamond Jim." The story of his gift is well known: Young successfully operated on Brady's prostate and in return received a gift to endow a new building.

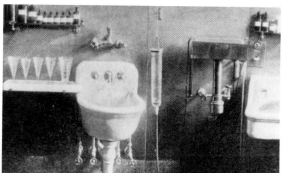

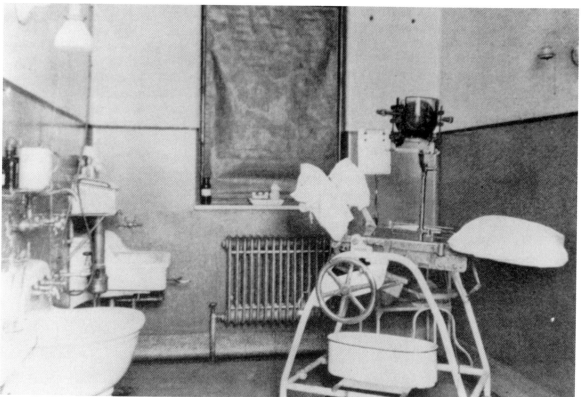

Treatment and examining rooms in the Brady Institute.

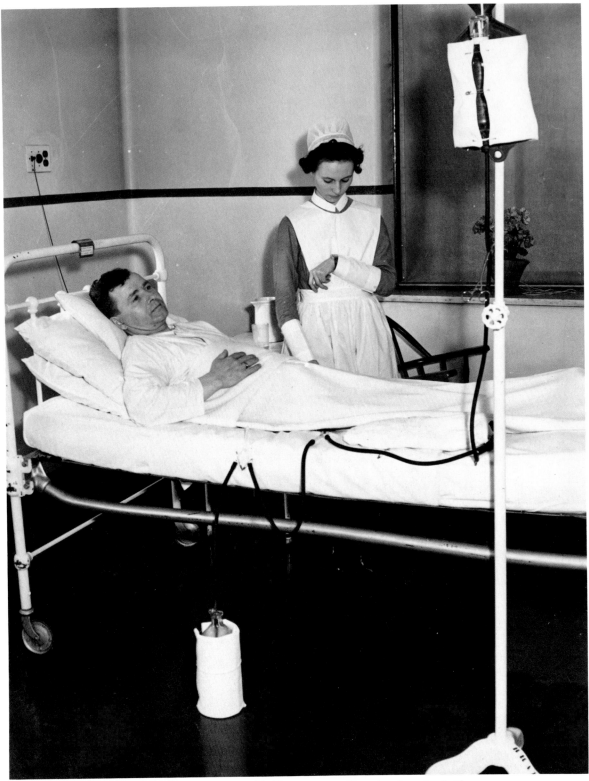

This photograph shows the technique of intermittent bladder irrigation. Note that the urine bottle on the floor is discreetly wrapped. The tubing is arranged in the typical Y-shaped manner.

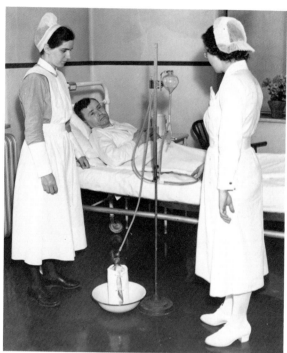

Apparatus for bladder decompression.

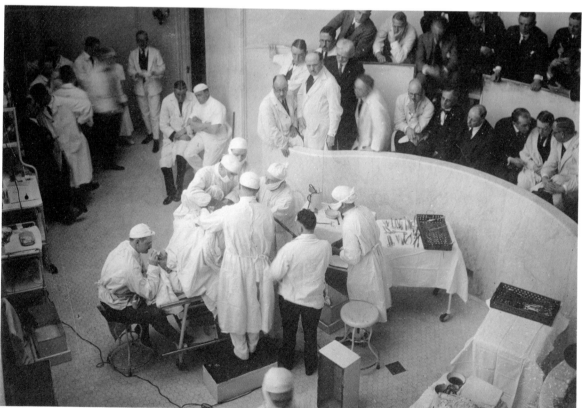

Hugh Young performing perineal prostatectomy, 1927.

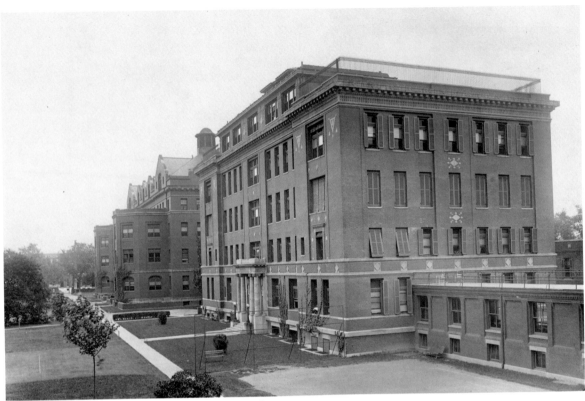

When the Harriet Lane Home opened in 1912, specialty hospitals for children were not yet a common feature of the American medical scene. According to L. Emmett Holt, a pioneer in pediatrics and the mentor of Johns Hopkins' first full-time pediatrician-in-chief, John Howland, only twenty-two American cities at that time had children's hospitals.

As a legal entity, the Harriet Lane Home for Invalid Children dated back to 1883. The trustees of that endowment in 1906 decided to enter into an agreement with the Johns Hopkins Hospital to construct a building on the south side of the hospital lot. This five-story structure, with three pavilions at its rear, was completed in 1912.

The main building was designed for the care of children with noninfectious illnesses. The west pavilion housed patients with scarlet fever, and diphtheria was treated in the east pavilion. This arrangement not only attests to the acceptance of the theory of disease transmission, but also affords an indication of the diseases prevalent among children at the time. The middle pavilion was used for an observation period until a proper diagnosis was made, with the hope that the main hospital would thereby be kept free from epidemics.

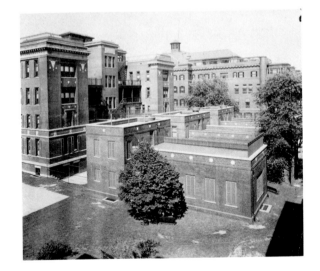

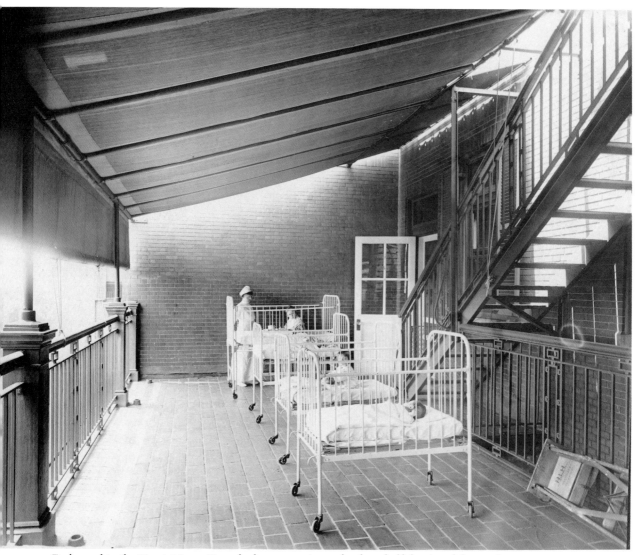

Each ward in the Harriet Lane Home had an open-air porch, about half the size of the ward itself. The beds were fitted with large casters so that they could be moved easily.

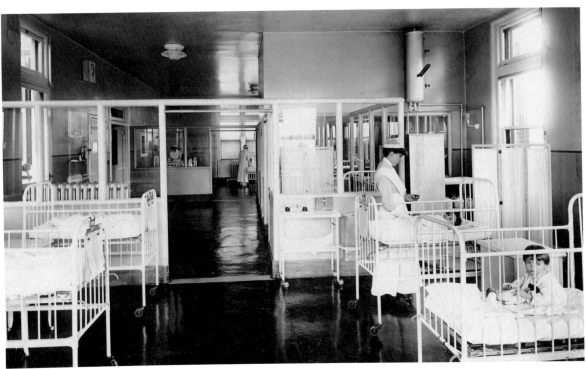

The Harriet Lane wards had minimal artificial lighting but ample windows, and to enhance brightness, the interior finish was deliberately maintained in light colors.

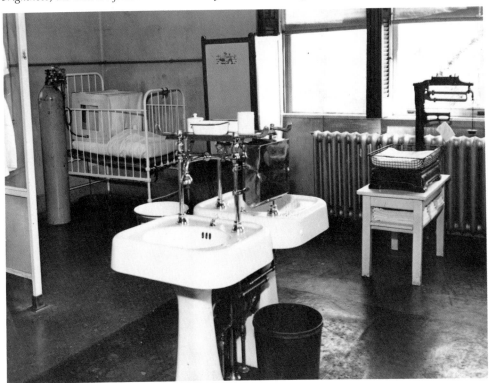

Note the oxygen tent and the double sink equipped with large faucet handles, which could be moved by an elbow or upper arm and thus did not require the use of the nurse's hands.

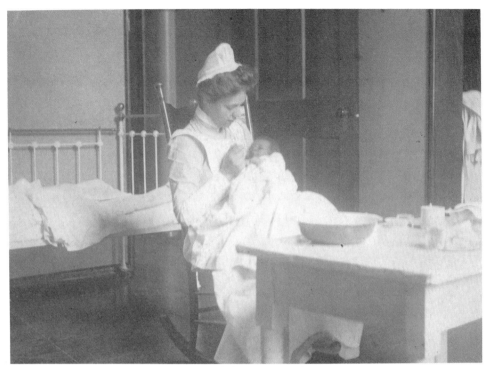

Feeding babies in the hospital, at the turn of the century and in 1977. By 1977, some of the work formerly done by nurses had been taken over by nurses' aides. Despite the revolution in equipment and service devoted to the newborn, the rocking chair remains part of good pediatric care at Hopkins.

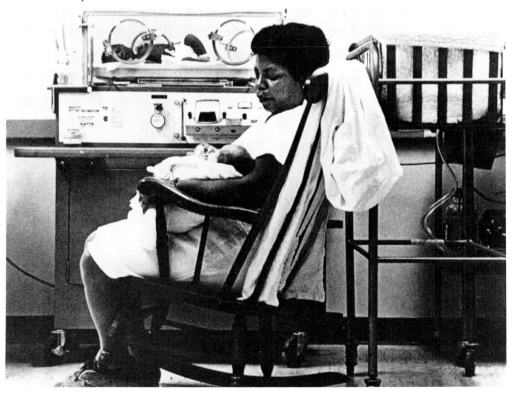

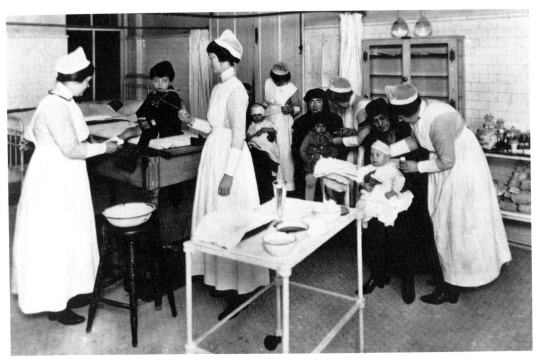

Then, as now, the outpatient department of the Harriet Lane Home was the scene of much of the activity. The photograph of nurses bandaging or rebandaging children in the clinic dates from the early 1920s. The crowded waiting room was a typical scene of the 1930s and 1940s.

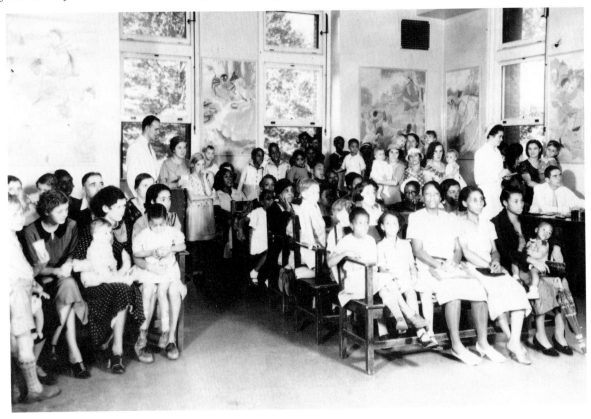

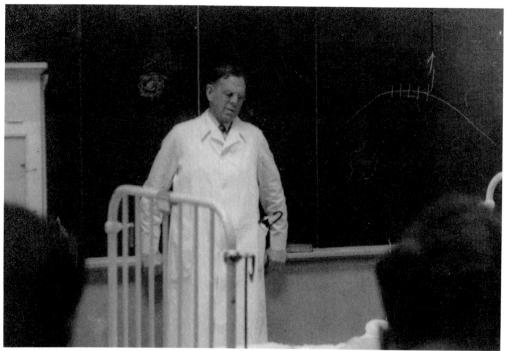

Clinical instruction at the bedside, conducted in the teaching room at the rear of the Harriet Lane Home, by Edwards A. Park, director of the Department of Pediatrics from 1927 to 1946.

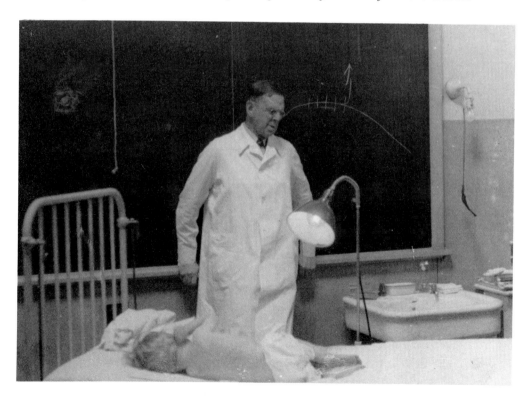

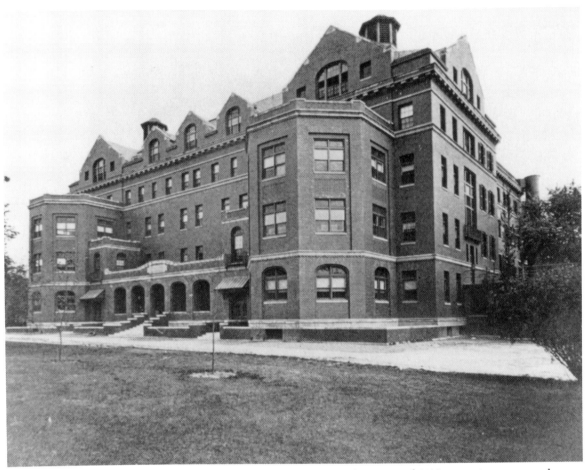

The opening of the Henry Phipps Psychiatric Clinic in April 1913 was as important to the general field of psychiatry as it would be for the hospital and school of medicine. The Phipps Clinic was situated immediately east of the new Harriet Lane Home. With the opening of this large new facility, Meyer capitalized on his opportunities.

Both the interior and the grounds of the Phipps Clinic were particularly designed to provide pleasant surroundings for patients. The careful attention to architectural detail is depicted in the pen-and-ink sketch made in 1932 by a long-time Phipps ward attendant, Lawrence Emge.

Both for teaching and in order to shape a really useful plant which could be a model of service to any locality or community, it was essential to provide facilities for the admission of any type of mental disorder from the very lightest to the gravest forms, which formerly were thrust into jails and lock-ups until they could be transferred to the padded rooms or cells of the asylums. It is among these cases that the greatest number of unnecessary deaths and abuses do take place, and it is absolutely essential that medical students and physicians trying to get acquainted with psychiatry must have an opportunity to learn to handle these cases and the situations they involve in the best possible manner. What we need in psychiatry is not an additional emphasis of the idea of stigma and contrast between special hospitals and the asylums but an assurance to the public that cases with mental disorders, no matter how slight or no matter how grave, can find proper care and treatment in modern hospitals.

—Adolf Meyer[13]

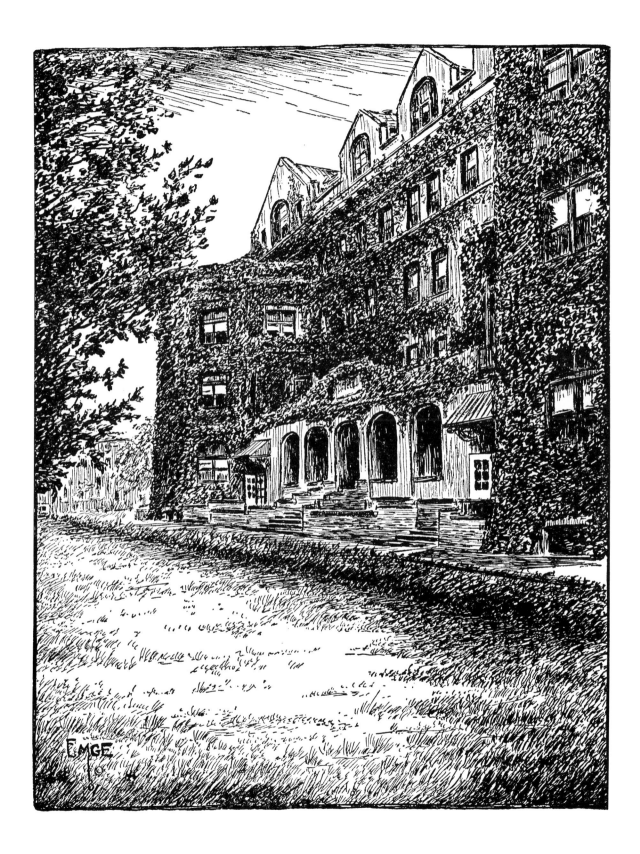

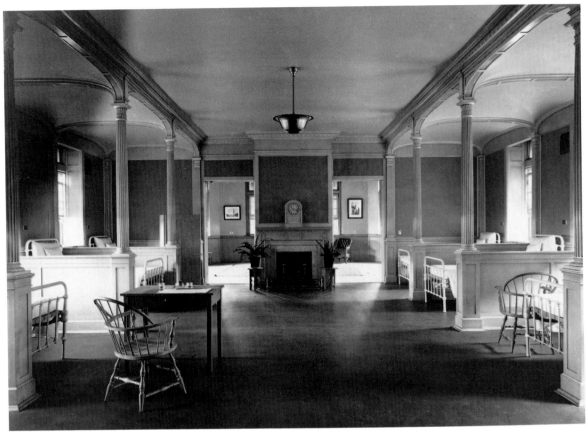

This view of what was called a "semi-quiet" ward was taken soon after the Phipps Clinic opened. As the accompanying quotation reveals, the word quiet *referred not to the surroundings but to the patients.*

For the . . . hospital division we have to provide an admission ward; facilities for the care of specially excited cases; then a semi-quiet ward; a quiet ward; and a special ward for such cases as one would not care to bring into contact with the more decidedly mental disorders or mentally disturbed patients.

—Adolf Meyer[14]

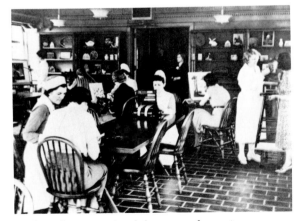

Facilities for occupational therapy and exercise.

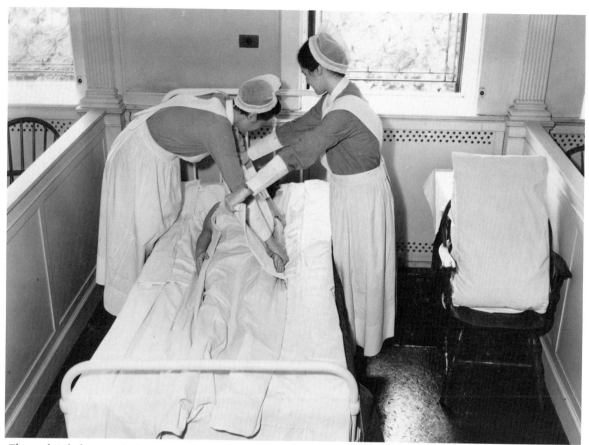

This undated photograph shows two Phipps Clinic nurses applying a sedative pack.

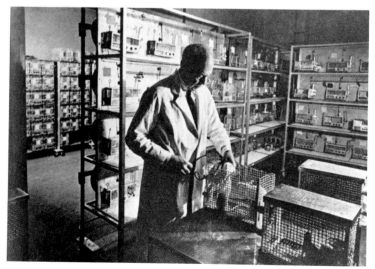

Curt P. Richter developed the Psychobiology Laboratory in the Phipps Institute, succeeding his mentor, John B. Watson.

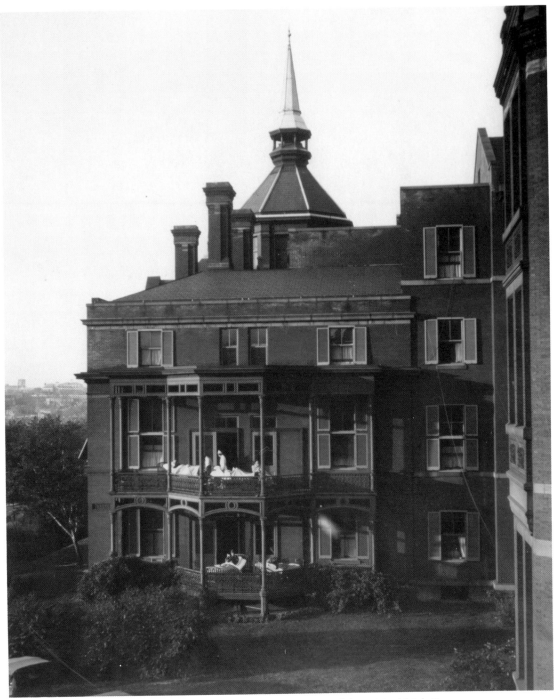

The Marburg Memorial Building, for private patients, an extension of the original Male Pay Ward, was built with funds donated by the family of Charles L. Marburg.

With the opening of three large hospital buildings in the same year—the Harriet Lane Clinic, the Phipps Clinic, and the Marburg Building—Hopkins experienced a sudden shortage of accommodations for nurses. The Trustees therefore decided to renovate the original women's private ward as temporary additional residence space for nurses.

A large doctor's dining room was located adjacent to the Marburg Building until the early 1960s, when it was demolished to make room for the Children's Medical and Surgical Center.

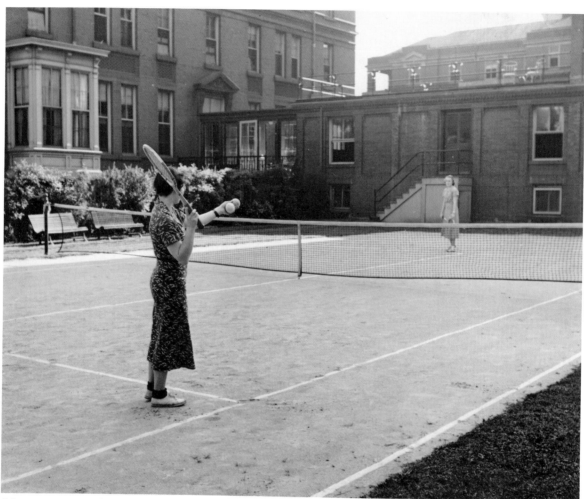

Many generations of nurses and Hopkins physicians used the tennis court between the Gynecological Building (later the Wilmer Institute) and the Harriet Lane Home. The building on the left is the Nurses' Home; beyond the courts are the Bridge and the Gynecological Building.

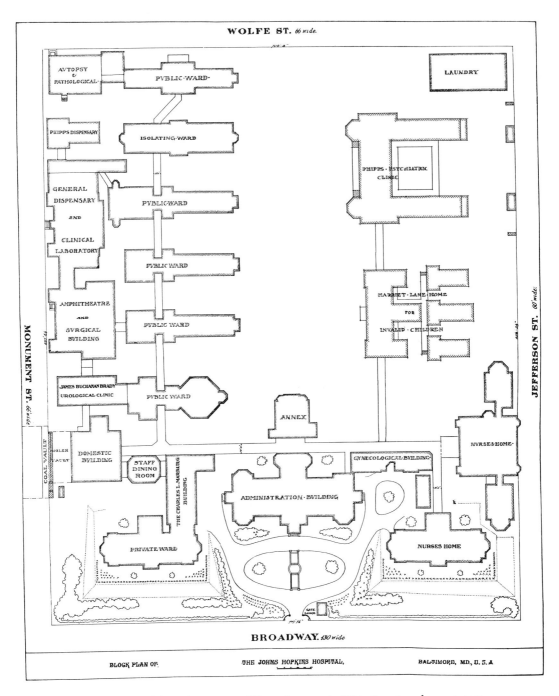

By the time the hospital celebrated its twenty-fifth anniversary in 1914, its outward appearance had changed extensively, as a comparison of the block plans of 1890 (on pp. 10–11) and 1914 shows. By 1914, the open space on the south side of the hospital lot was filled. The space had been bare because funds were not available to construct the planned mirror-image wards, but now it was occupied by buildings for the developing fields of pediatrics and psychiatry. It was thus used for a type of growth that the original planners could not have envisioned. What was at first a disadvantage—the absence of the symmetrical row of wards—later gave the hospital the flexibility to construct buildings for the future.

4

THE BUILDING BOOM OF THE 1920s

Although the model of Johns Hopkins medicine was well established by 1914, in subsequent decades both the hospital and medical school buildings continued to grow larger and more elaborate. Between the end of World War I and the onset of the worldwide depression of the early 1930s, a dozen new or replacement buildings appeared. New hospital facilities included a Woman's Clinic, a new outpatient building, modern clinics for medicine and surgery, an ophthalmology center, a new amphitheater, and new quarters for nurses. The medical school acquired a more suitable space for pathology, physiological chemistry, and —at last—a proper library that would serve as a central resource for both the medical school and the hospital.

Once the original buildings were in use, subsequent construction seems to have followed no master plan. Responses to unexpected opportunities and to the needs of individual departments governed the building boom of the 1920s. With rare exceptions, such as the Phipps Psychiatric Clinic and the Welch Library, Hopkins achieved far more distinction in medicine, public health, and research than it did in architectural design or spatial unity on the East Baltimore campus.

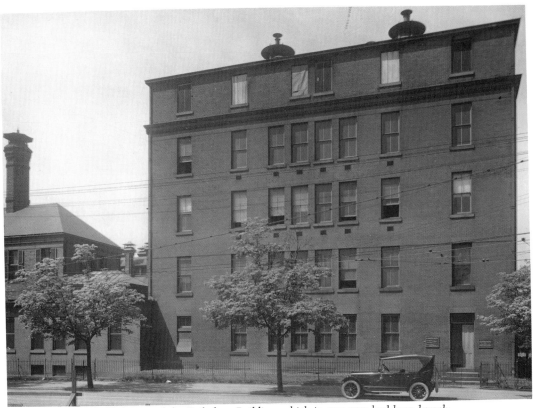

A fire in January 1920 destroyed the Pathology Building, which in any case had been largely outgrown. A gift of $400,000 from the Rockefeller Foundation and an additional $200,000 from university endowment funds enabled the start of construction of a new building in early 1922. The eight-story building, whose top floor originally contained animal rooms, was completed later the following year, and it still stands on the corner of Monument and Wolfe streets.

Above, the old Pathology Building shortly before it burned down.

Below, the completed new building, with the one-story autopsy room, Woman's Clinic, and Phipps Psychiatric Clinic beyond.

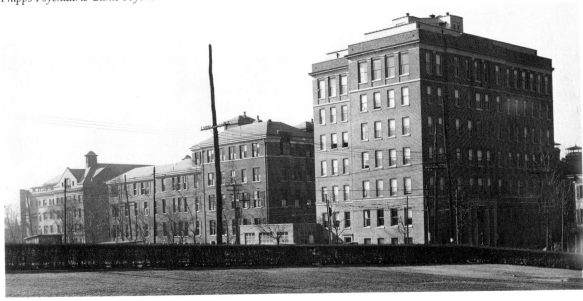

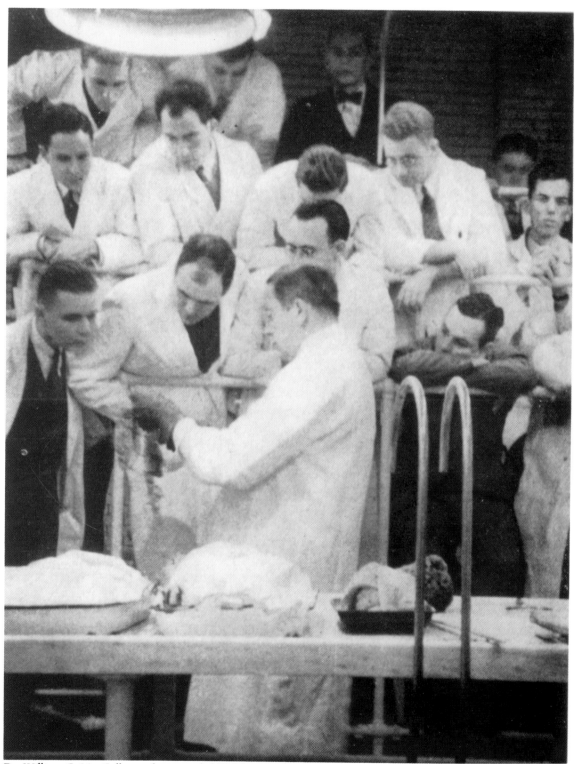

Dr. William G. MacCallum, who succeeded Welch as professor of pathology, is shown here demonstrating gross specimens (taken ca. 1930). MacCallum was both a gifted investigator and an excellent teacher.

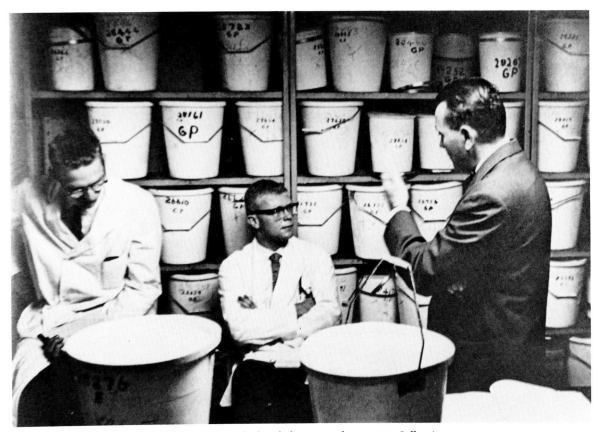

Generations of second-year medical students studied pathology according to MacCallum's textbook, first published in 1916. Diseased organs, in white buckets, were arranged in separate rooms in the order in which they were discussed in MacCallum's book. As students finished one section, they would move on to the next set of buckets.

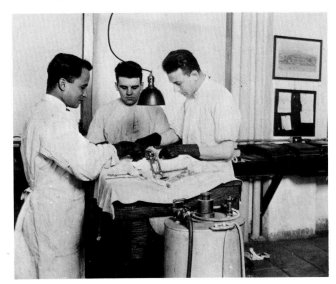

Arnold R. Rich, who succeeded MacCallum as chairman of the Department of Pathology, is shown at work in his laboratory. Note the comparative simplicity of his equipment.

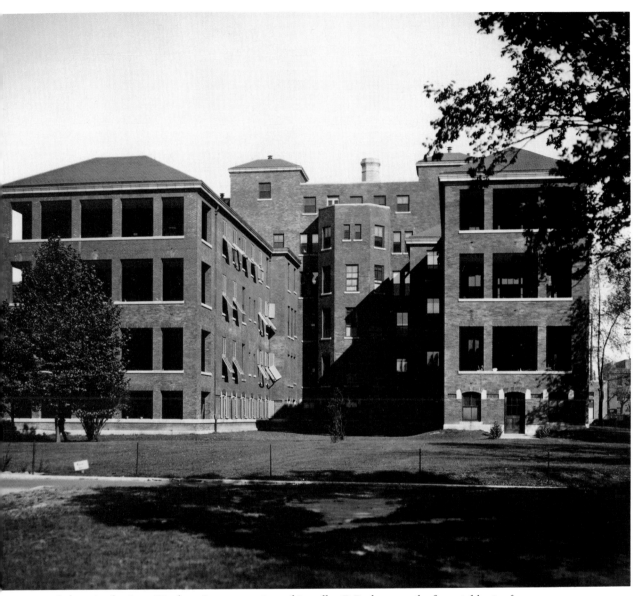

A donation by Lucy Wortham James, a patient of Lewellys F. Barker, was the financial basis of the Woman's Clinic, which was opened in 1922. Its five floors contained sixty obstetrical beds and sixty-six gynecological beds, ten private rooms for obstetrical patients, and seventeen cubicles for gynecological and obstetrical patients. (Private gynecological patients were accommodated in the Marburg Building.) A sixth floor was added to house the gynecological operating rooms, which were constructed only after some protest from Thomas S. Cullen, director of the Department of Gynecology, and his staff, who felt that their operating rooms should be associated with the facilities of the Department of Surgery.

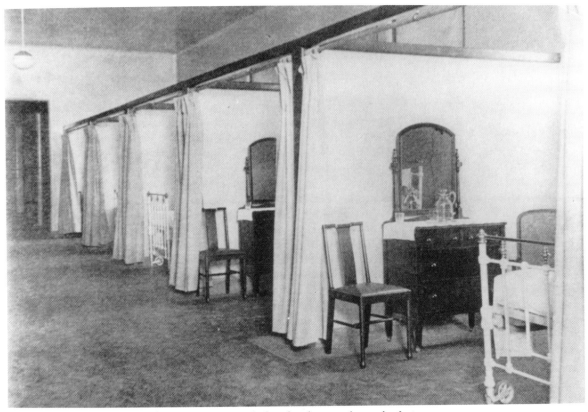

The photographs on this page show semi-private cubicles; the photographs on the facing page show wards in the Woman's Clinic. In contrast to the ward scenes shown in section 1, by this time wards offered patients the possibility of some privacy.

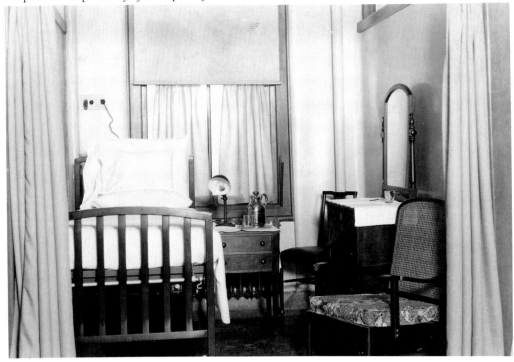

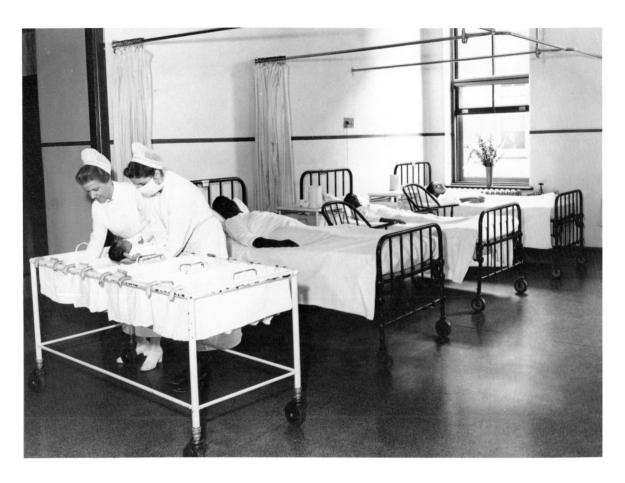

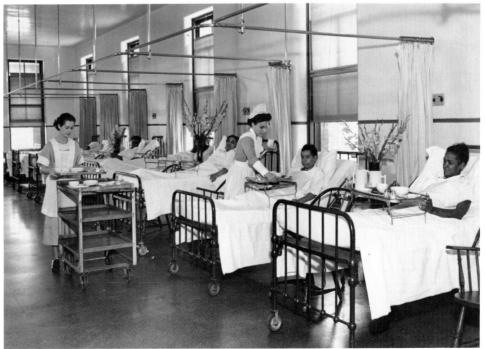

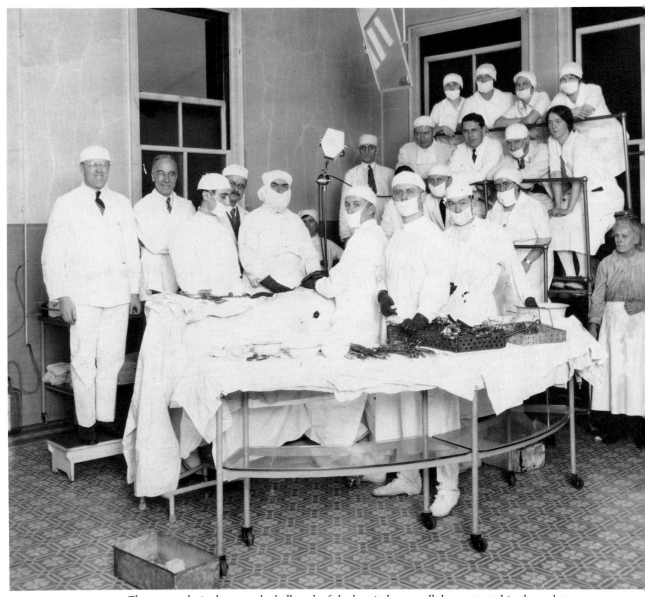

The camaraderie that was the hallmark of the hospital was well demonstrated in these photographs, taken at the time of the last operation in the old Gynecological Operating Room (on Saturday, January 22, 1927) and of the first in the department's new, larger quarters in the Woman's Clinic.

"Katie," who cleaned the room, was considered a sufficiently important part of the staff to be included in the photograph (above). Note the more solidly constructed platform for observers in the new operating room. In both operating room scenes, masks were still worn improperly, below the nose.

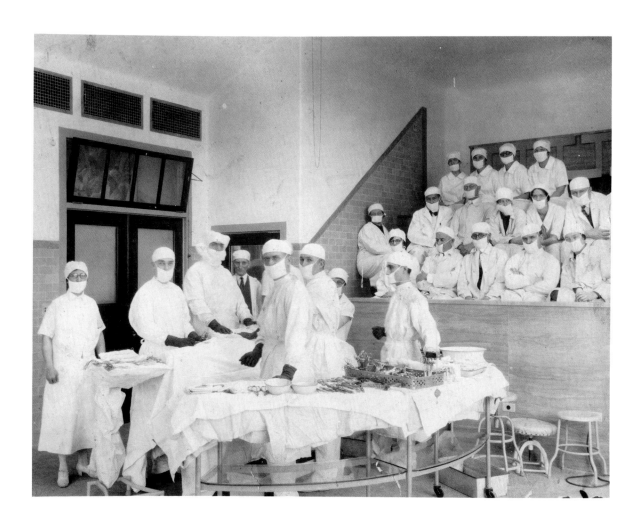

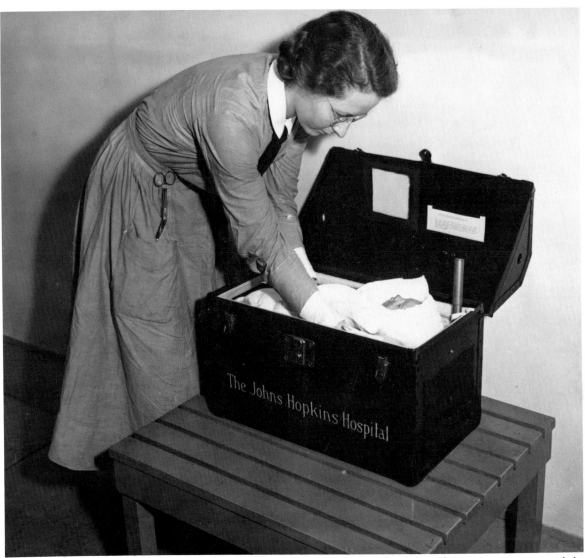

Not all the medical care occurred on the wards or in the clinics. The nursing service provided
help with home deliveries.

    In the second decade of this century, the hospital began to operate its own ambulance, a
1920s version of which is shown here (opposite, above), standing near its garage in the old
Dispensary Building.

    Social services also had a car for making home visits (opposite, below).

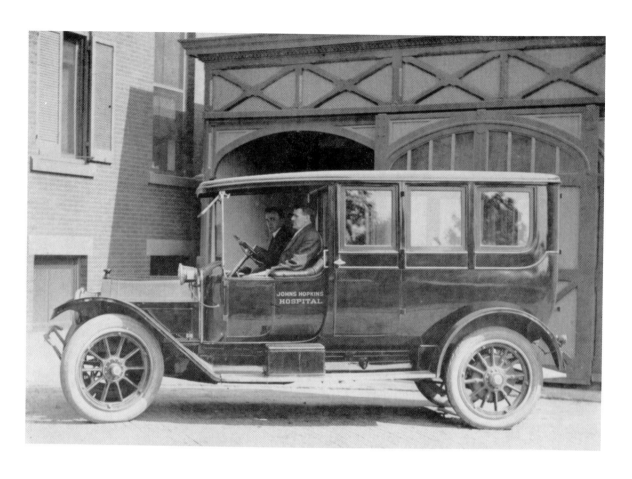

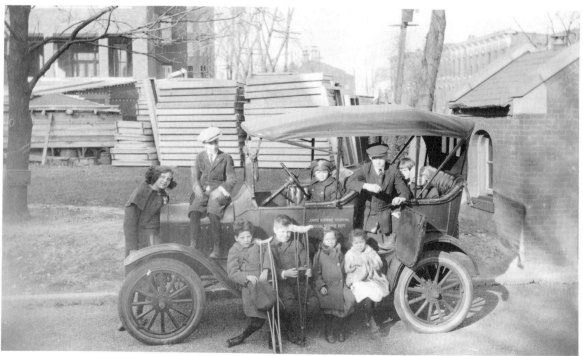

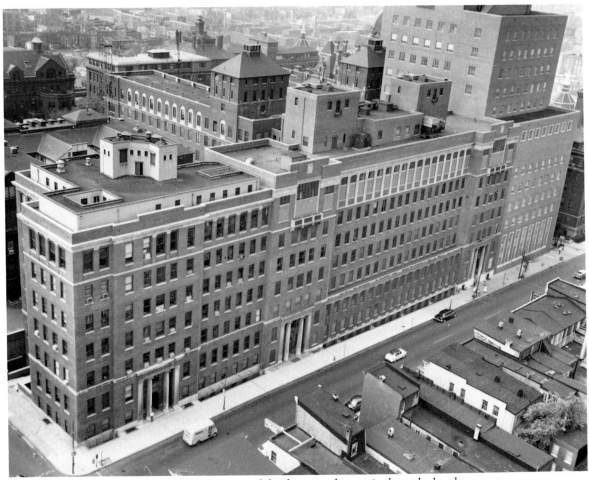

The name of Andrew Carnegie was as important to philanthropic endeavors in the early decades of the twentieth century as it was to America's industrial growth at the end of the previous one. Carnegie the steel magnate was also the Carnegie of the Foundation for the Advancement of Teaching, which provided funds for pensions for college teachers and underwrote many studies of professions in America, including the well-known 1910 report on medical education by Abraham Flexner.

In 1923, Henry S. Pritchett, acting president of the parent Carnegie Corporation, informed University President Frank J. Goodnow that two million dollars was to be given to Johns Hopkins to build a dispensary.

The Dispensary, given the Carnegie name, opened in 1927; a wide variety of activities took place in the building, as portrayed in the photographs that follow.

The Carnegie Building extends along Monument Street between the Pathology Building on the corner of Wolfe Street and the Blalock Building, constructed later to the west (at the right in the photograph).

The trustees [of the Carnegie Corporation] have made this grant in recognition of the important part which the Johns Hopkins Medical School has played in the development of scientific medicine, and more particularly in the hope that what was orginally planned as an out-patient department primarily for the instruction of young physicians and surgeons may become, under the enlarged plan which you have adopted, a diagnostic clinic offering to those of modest means the facilities of modern medical science, and having a close cooperation with the medical practitioners to whom such patients now resort. The trustees also hope that the dispensary and clinic thus established may be closely related to the School of Hygiene which is to be situated in a building just across the street, and that the influence upon the persons who may resort to the Clinic may be representative no less of the prevention than of the cure of disease. It is our anticipation that this enterprise may develop into a fruitful and far-reaching agency in medical education and practice, and that it may serve to lead the way to a feasible method by which the great mass of persons living in cities upon moderate incomes may be brought into relation with the best results and practices of modern medicine.

The trustees venture to add, although they never attach conditions involving the perpetuation of names of individuals, they would be pleased if this new building might bear an inscription setting forth the warm regard that Mr. Carnegie had for President Gilman and the appreciation which Mr. Carnegie held for the advice and assistance that he rendered in the establishment of the Carnegie Institute of Washington.

—Henry S. Pritchett[1]

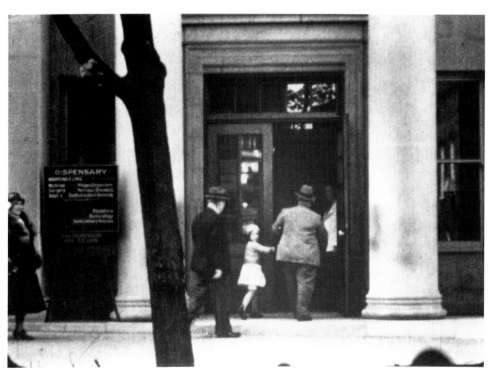

Patients at the main entrance to the Carnegie Building, ca. 1930.

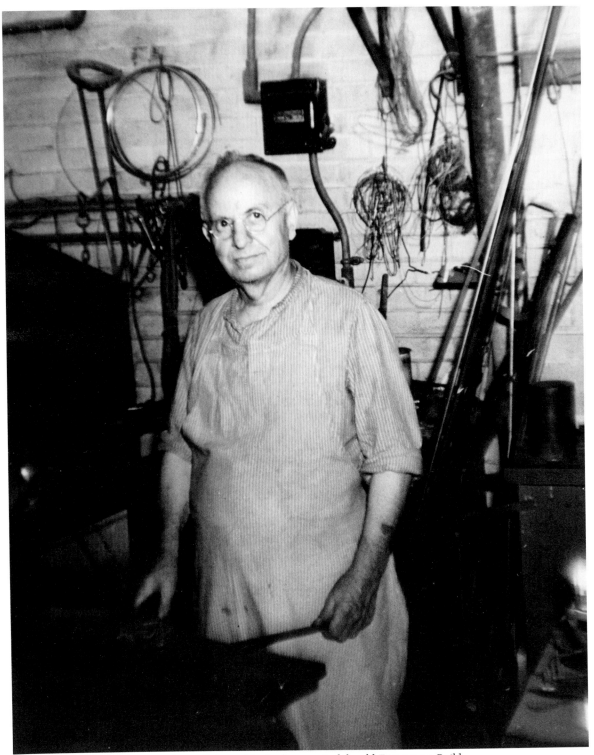

The Orthopedic Brace Shop was formerly located in the basement of the old Dispensary Building. This 1942 photograph shows brace-maker Chris Hupfeld with his tools.

The new medical dispensary was planned along novel lines. The traditional large, crowded waiting room was replaced with several smaller units, with space for twenty-five to forty patients, in the section of the building occupied by the Department of Medicine. The second, third, and fourth floors contained the several medical clinics; teaching units, to each of which were assigned eight students, were located in these clinics.

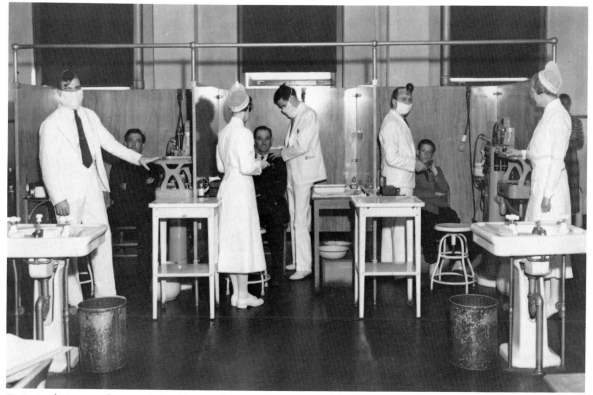

Patients, doctors, and nurses in the Nose and Throat Dispensary of the Carnegie Building.

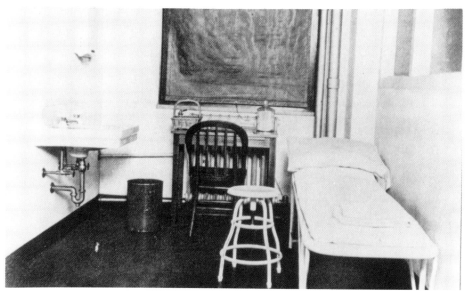

A typical examining room for medical patients in the Carnegie Dispensary.

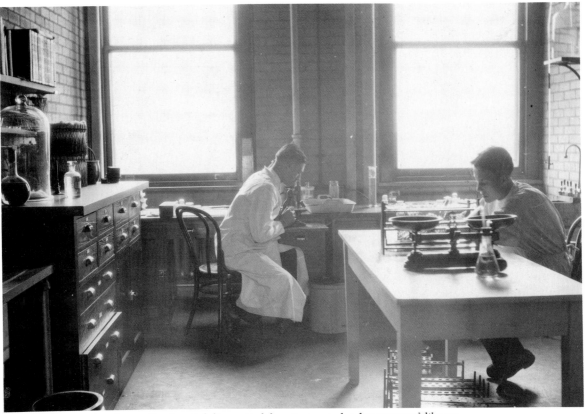

Research laboratories, the routine hospital diagnostic laboratories, and a departmental library were located on the fifth and sixth floors.

Above, one of these research laboratories assigned to the Department of Medicine.

Below, the laboratory for instruction in clinical microscopy, which replaced Osler's facility for that purpose when the Carnegie was built. Note the addition of running water and chemical hoods.

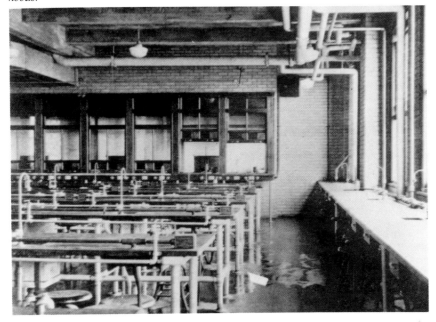

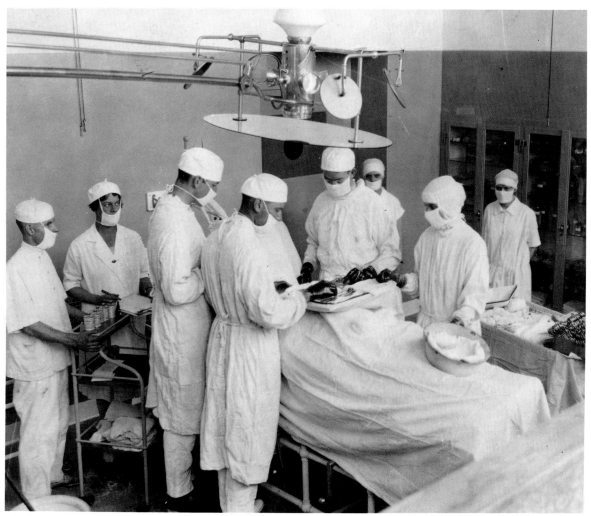

This was the first operation performed in the Carnegie's new operating rooms, on August 27, 1927. The surgeon, on the far side of the table, is William F. Rienhoff. The taller of the two assistants is Deryl Hart, who in 1930 became the first chairman of surgery at Duke University, and in the early 1950s the president of Duke.

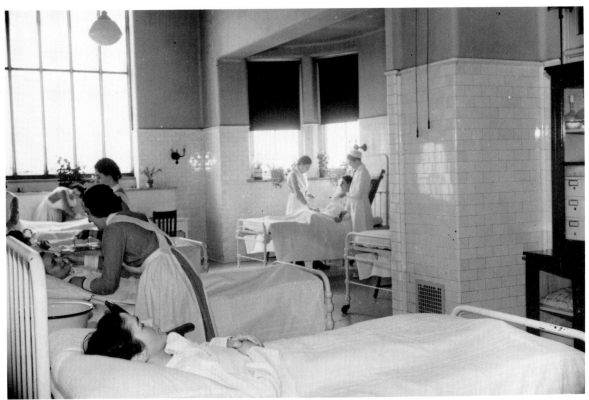

When the operating rooms were moved to the Carnegie Building, the area they occupied in the old Surgical Building was converted to teaching space for the school of nursing.

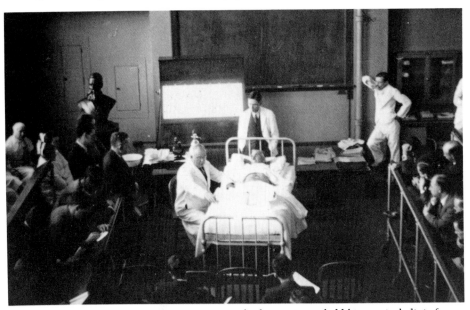

The seventh-floor classroom, where Surgeon-in-Chief Dean Lewis held his surgical clinic for medical students each Friday. Lewis was a dramatic teacher whose pedagogical technique created widespread apprehension among the students present. Lewis picked students at random to descend from the stands to the bedside. There, they underwent his sharp questioning concerning the patient at hand.

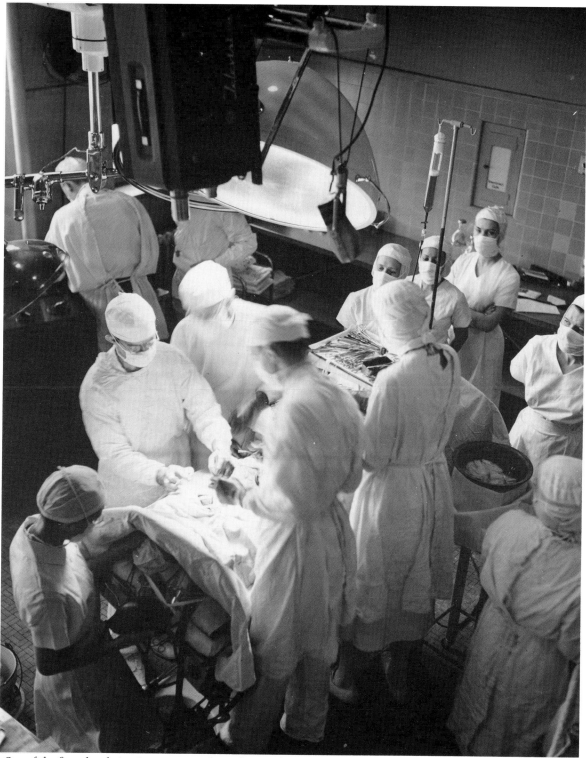

One of the first closed-circuit operations televised at Hopkins was this "blue-baby" procedure performed in the Carnegie by Alfred Blalock on February 28, 1947. The assistant directly across the table is Henry Bahnson.

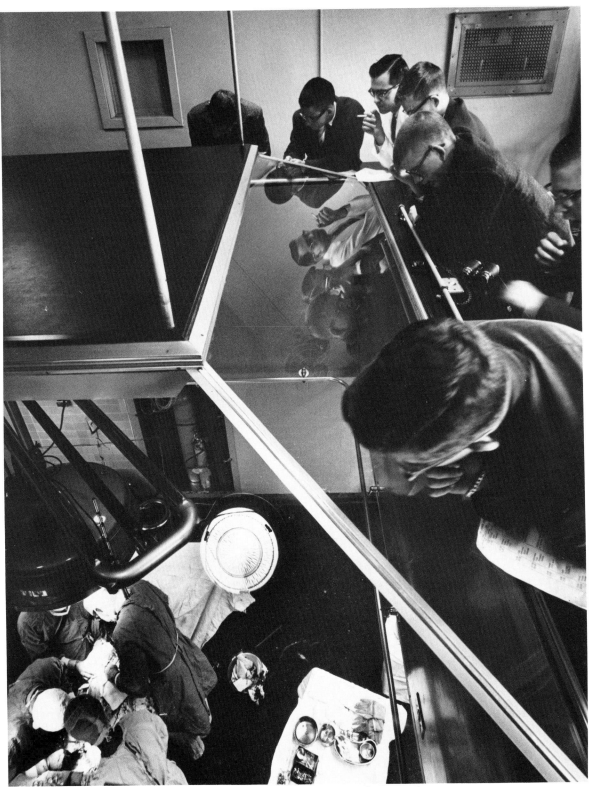

Students observing an operation in the Carnegie in 1958 were comparatively remote from the scene.

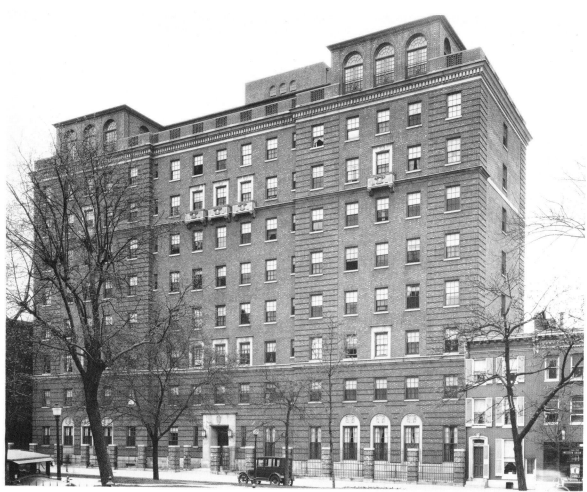

Hampton House, named for Isabel Hampton, the first superintendent of nurses, opened as a residence in 1926. It had single rooms for 235, and suites for members of the nursing school staff.

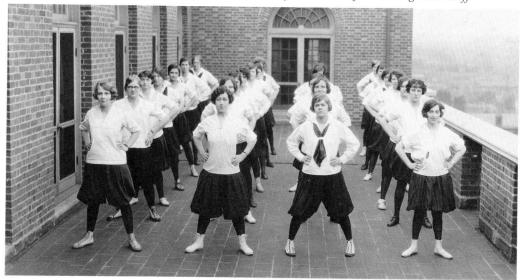

The roof of Hampton House was the scene of classes in "body mechanics."

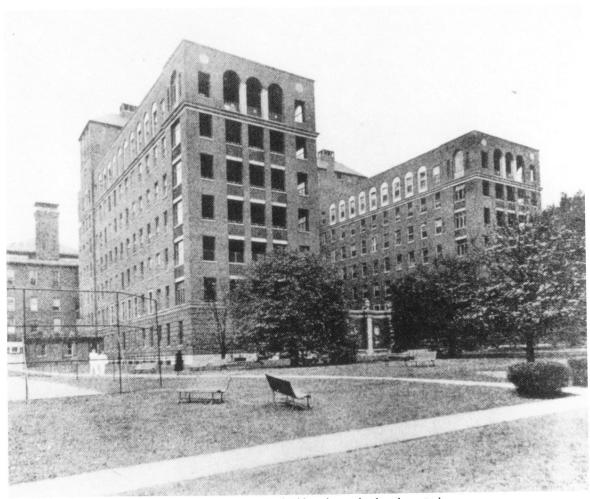

Early in the 1920s, funds were raised to construct a new building for medical and surgical patients. The Osler and Halsted clinics opened a decade later, in 1931. The building consisted of two symmetrical wings of seven stories each, replacing the old wards D, E, F, G, M, and O. A ground floor amphitheater was added between the wings and named in honor of Dr. Henry M. Hurd, superintendent for the first twenty-two years of the hospital's existence.

Warfield T. Longcope, the professor of medicine, spoke at the dedication of the three buildings in 1932. In his address, he pointed out that the completion of the new building placed the three essentials for teaching good medicine and surgery in close proximity: ambulatory patients in the clinic, inpatients on the wards, and ample laboratory facilities.

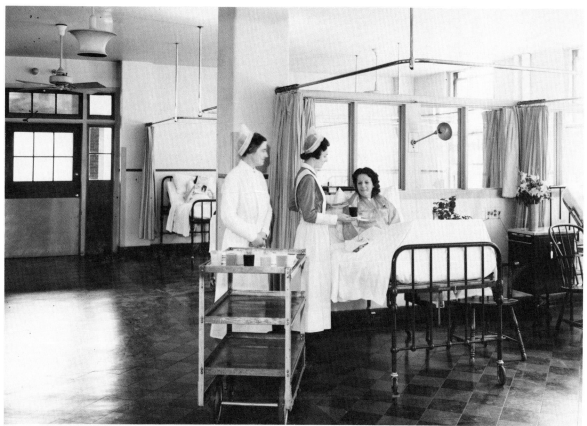

Typical scene on an Osler ward.

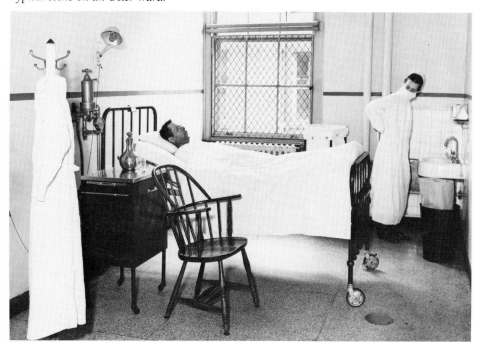

Single room, Osler men's ward. Critically ill patients occupied these rooms, which were located near the nurses' station, so that the patient could be closely observed.

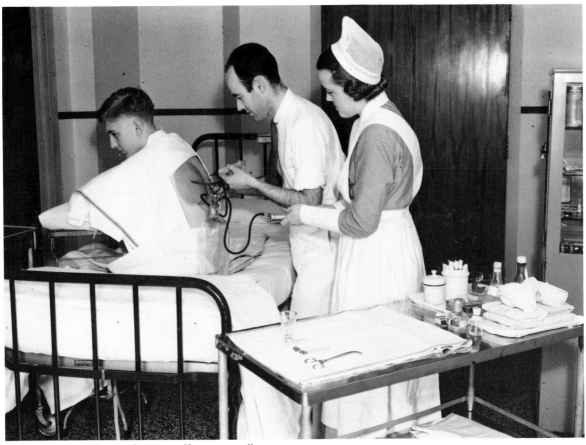

Chest drainage, Osler ward. House officer is Russell Williams, chief medical resident (Hopkins Class of 1934).

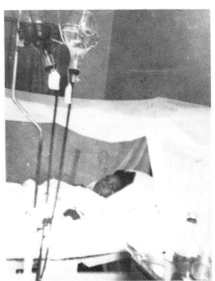

Treatment of typhoid fever. Patients with this disease were subject to sudden medical crises. The protective netting isolated the patient from others on the ward while allowing constant observation of the patient.

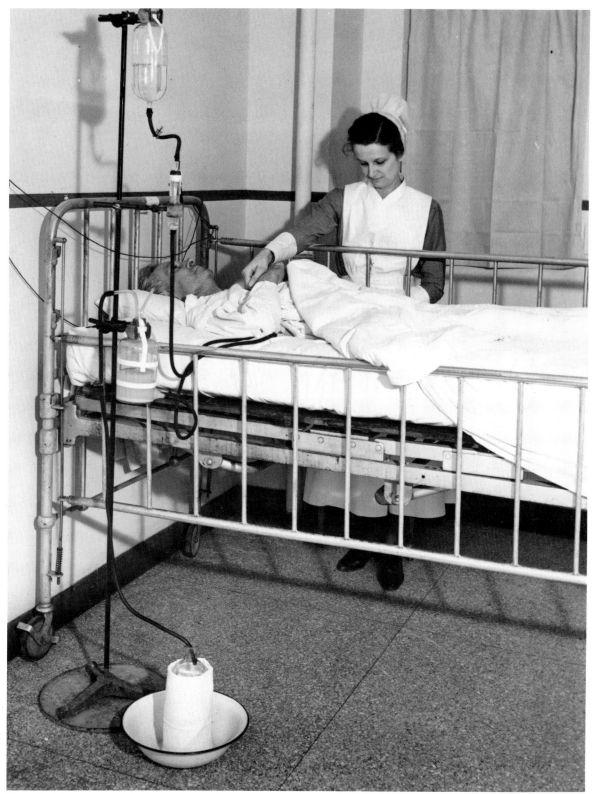

Hart tidal drainage used in the treatment of empyema.

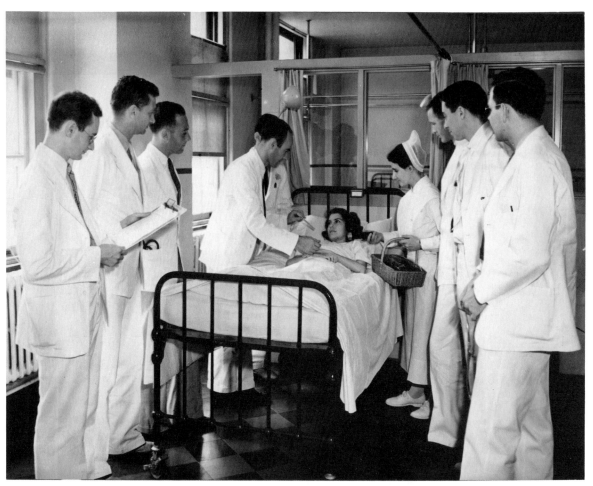

Morning rounds, Osler service.

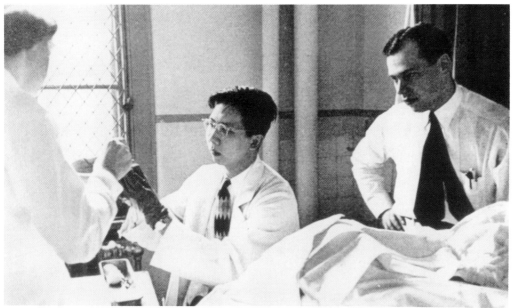

An intern on the Osler service supervising a fourth-year medical student who is performing a lumbar puncture.

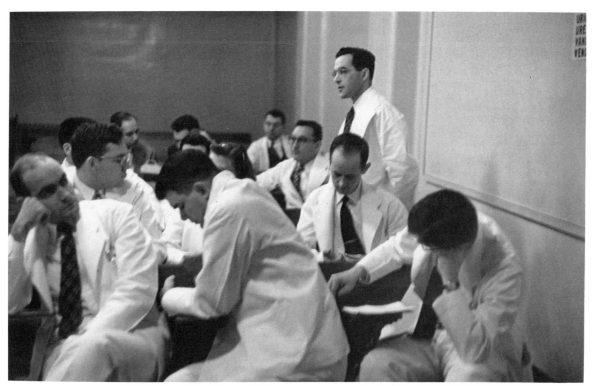

The chief resident is giving his customary teaching session at the end of the day to his weary resident staff. The resident is Sherman Mellinkoff, who became dean of the School of Medicine at the University of California at Los Angeles.

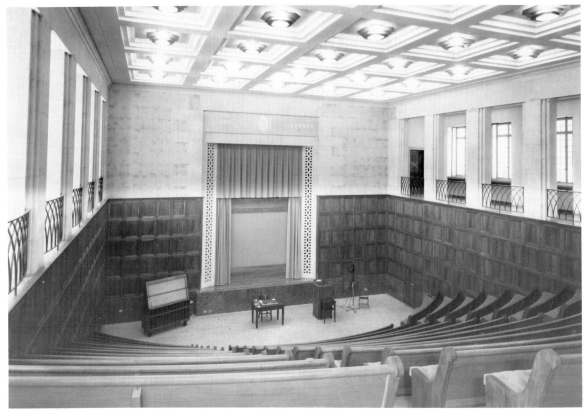

Henry M. Hurd Memorial Hall, opened in 1932, was the scene of many historic presentations. Here, in the first year of its use, Harvey Cushing described the syndrome that bears his name, and in 1945, Alfred Blalock and Helen B. Taussig reported the results of their new approach to the treatment of congenital heart disease.

Weekly staff rounds for the Department of Medicine were conducted by department chairman A. McGehee Harvey. Until 1946, rounds took place at the patient's bedside. When the group attending became too large, rounds were moved to Hurd Hall and the patients were brought in from the ward.

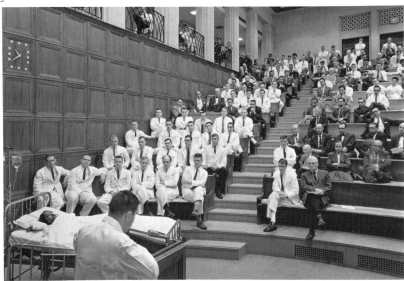

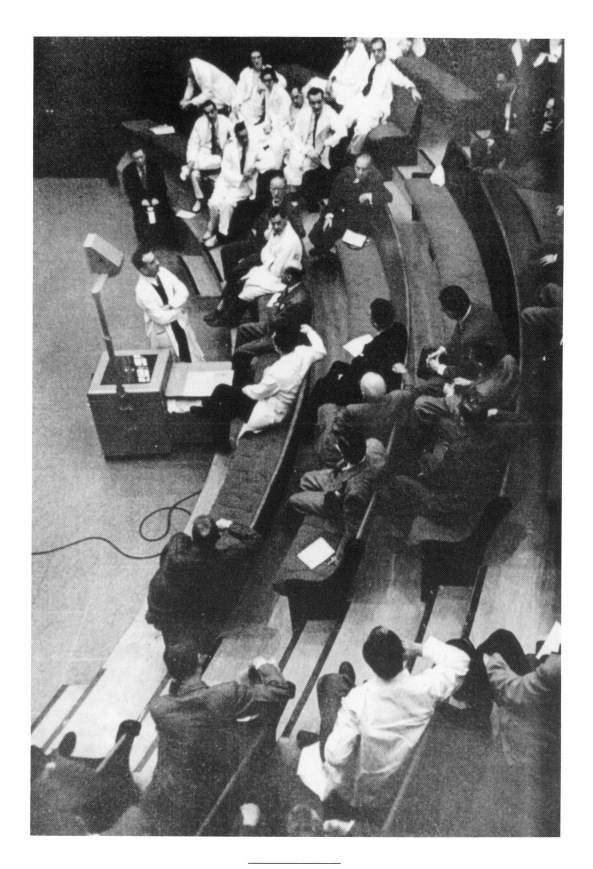

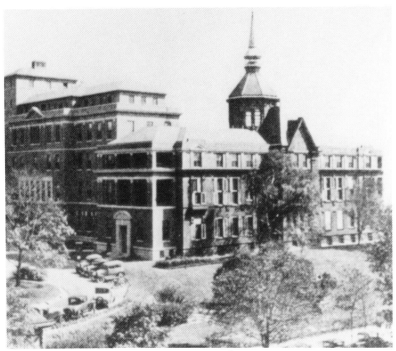

The Wilmer Ophthalmological Institute opened in 1925 with money raised from foundations
and from individual donors. The building, completed in 1928, was situated on the southwest
corner of the hospital lot. Its nearly 20,000 square feet of clinical and research space was fash-
ioned from the Female Pay Ward at the southwest corner of the hospital lot on Broadway.
Above, the Wilmer Institute in 1929; below, the original building with one of its additions, the
Alan C. Woods Research Building, in 1964 (see p. 158).

The old Gynecological Operating Room became a part of the Wilmer Institute (the entrance
lobby, which extended from the main corridor).

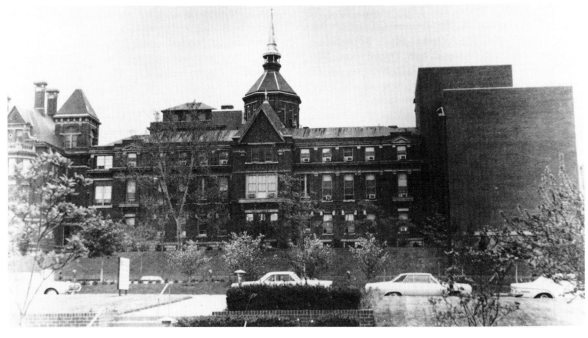

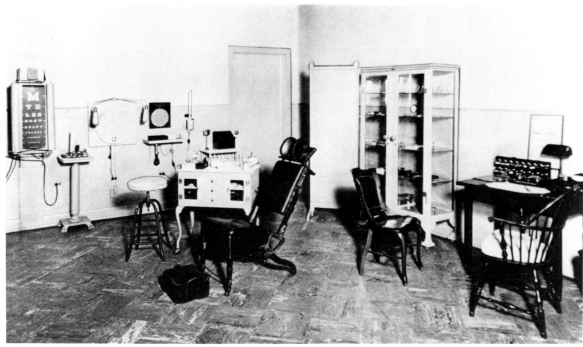

Wilmer's examining room and "The President's Chair."

Dr. Wilmer always had some warm, reassuring word to every new patient. He was seated at his desk, where the Senior Resident's history was amplified. . . . The examination was begun by moving the patient to the center of the room where he was seated in the "famous President's Chair." Many times Dr. Wilmer would comment, "This chair has held every President of the United States from McKinley to Franklin Roosevelt, so don't worry about leaning back. Just remember, it held President Taft when he weighed 350 pounds."
     —M. Elliott Randolph and Robert B. Welch[2]

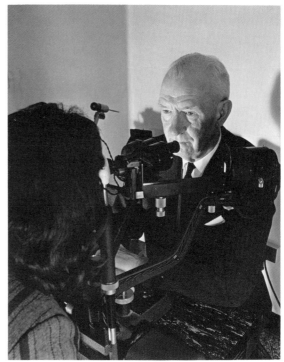

Frank B. Walsh, one of the great teachers trained by Wilmer, and a pioneer in the field of neuro-ophthalmology, is shown here measuring a patient's visual field.

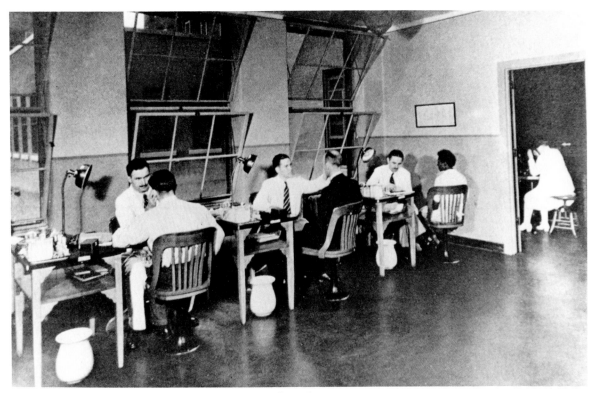

This is one of the two outpatient examination rooms in the Wilmer Institute in 1929.

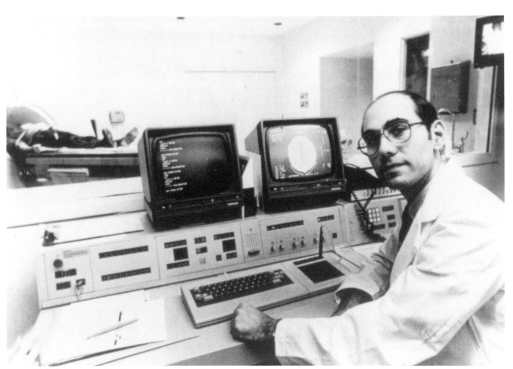

Faculty member Neil Miller performs a diagnostic procedure with the aid of computerized axial tomography in 1986.

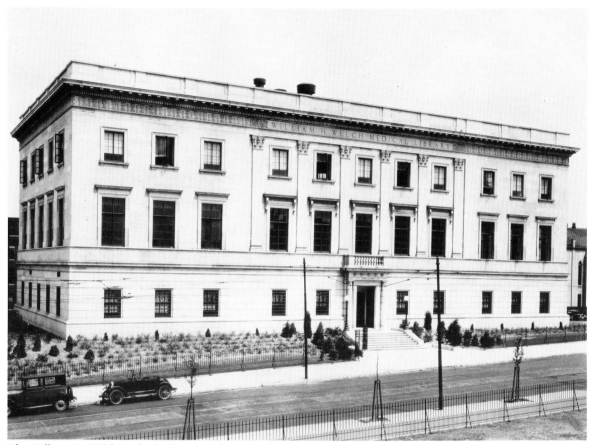

The William H. Welch Medical Library, dedicated in 1929 at its present site on the north side of Monument Street, between Wolfe and Washington streets, was designed to accommodate the libraries of the hospital, the school of hygiene, and the school of medicine. With eight levels of book stacks and three stories of reading rooms and offices, the handsome building was designed by the New York architect Edward L. Tilton in an Italian Renaissance style and was faced with variegated Indiana limestone. Within a decade it became one of the country's largest medical libraries.

From its beginnings, the Institute of the History of Medicine and its valuable collection of historical books has occupied the top (third) floor of the building.

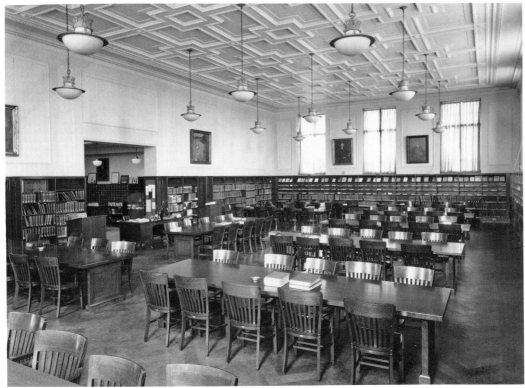

Above, the Library's Reading Room, now called the East Reading Room.

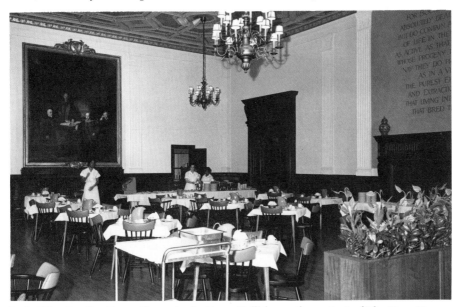

In the West Reading Room (formerly the Great Hall) hangs the portrait of The Four Doctors, *painted by John Singer Sargent in 1906. On the east wall hangs another Sargent portrait; while not as well known in the history of art, this painting of Mary Elizabeth Garrett is equally significant to the founding of the medical school, for it was through her generosity that the school could open its doors to its first small class in the autumn of 1893. In the 1960s, when the Children's Medical and Surgical Center was under construction, the Great Hall was used as a faculty club for lunch.*

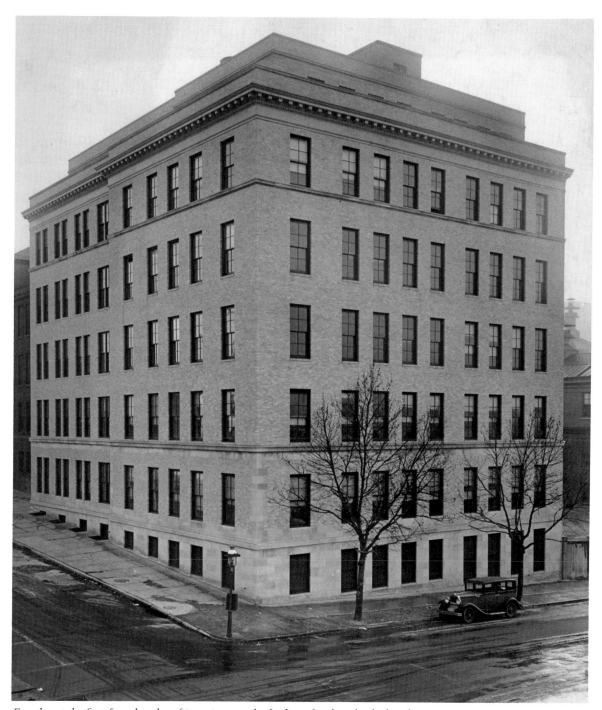

For almost the first four decades of its existence, the facilities for the school of medicine consisted of three buildings: the Women's Fund Memorial Building for anatomy, the Hunterian Laboratory, and the Physiology Building. In 1929, a new Physiology Building was constructed on the corner of Washington and Madison streets, providing much-needed space for the departments of Physiology, Pharmacology, and Physiological Chemistry. The top floor and part of the roof held animal quarters. The building was never formally named, but it came to be widely known as the "New Physiology Building," a designation dropped only when the original Physiology Building was demolished in 1959.

5

THE YEARS AFTER WORLD WAR II

Section 5 illustrates the changes in the Johns Hopkins Hospital and School of Medicine between 1930 and the present. The expansion of the medical school and hospital during these six decades has been mainly upwards, rather than outwards. Little has been added to the original tracts of land, and the hospital and medical school have thus been built and rebuilt on the same site. This process has sometimes required the demolition of cherished landmarks, such as the Women's Fund Memorial Building, which in the mid-1980s was replaced by the Preclinical Teaching Building. In an era of low-bid architecture, few of the buildings erected after World War II have been as architecturally distinguished as their predecessors.

The contents of the new buildings—facilities for patient care, teaching, and research—reflect one of the most prominent changes of the past six decades: the advance of technology. So substantial have these changes been that photographs of equipment from the 1950s look as distant from today as those of equipment from fifty years before.

The medical school's archives contains many photographs from the past six decades, but modern equipment and buildings can be found in medical schools across the country, and these pictures show Hopkins less specifically than do the pictures of the early years. It is the scenes of student life and the photographs that depict the traditions of Osler and the other original faculty as extended to modern times that remain as characteristic of Johns Hopkins today as they were a century ago.

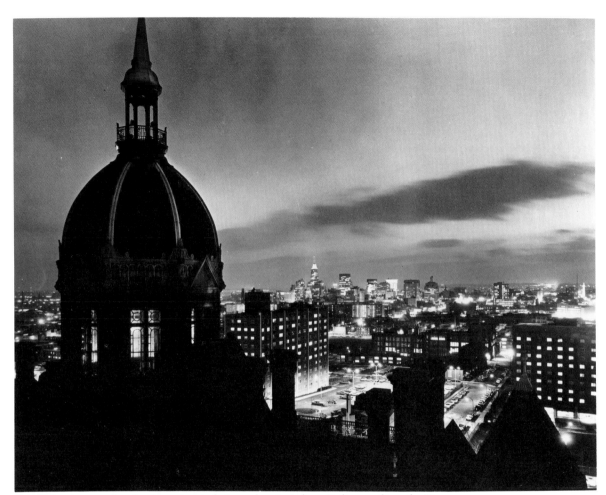

A twilight picture, taken by the eminent photographer A. Aubrey Bodine, outlines the Dome and depicts Hopkins as a vital part of Baltimore.

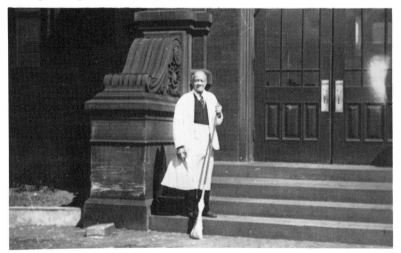

From the hospital's opening in 1889 (as legend has it) to the 1950s, William Thomas greeted all who came through the front door. This photograph was taken in the spring of 1949.

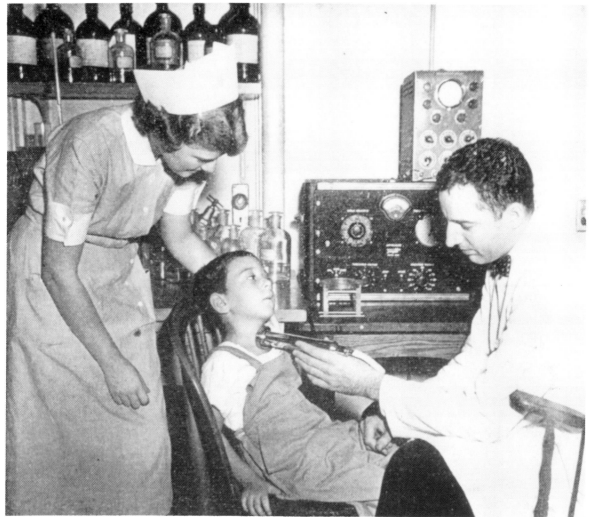

William Thomas's tenure spanned a time of great technological growth in the history of medicine. These advances were applied to all aspects of medicine at Johns Hopkins, particularly patient care and research.

   As an example, new diagnostic equipment became available to study the thyroid gland in the years immediately after World War II. In this photograph, a pediatrician, John F. Crigler, Jr., uses a Geiger counter to determine the activity of a young patient's thyroid gland. The child has taken a dose of radioactive iodine, and the Geiger counter will reveal its concentration in the thyroid.

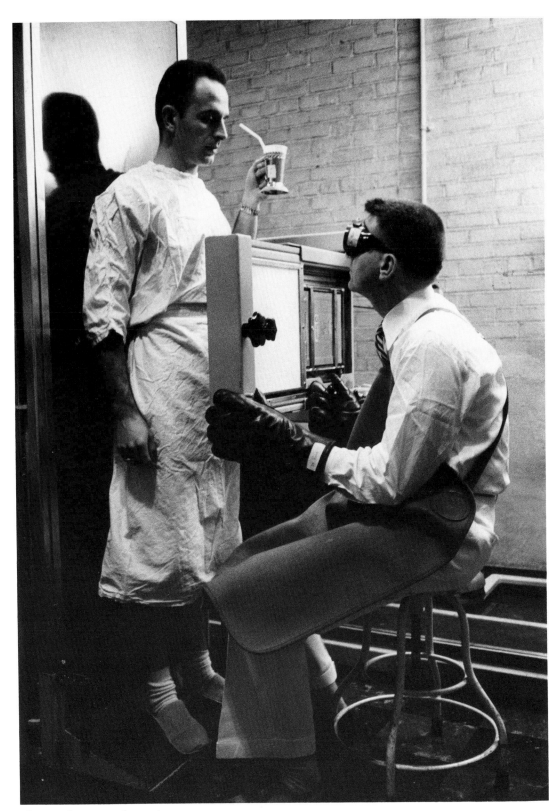

The use of x-rays in diagnosis.

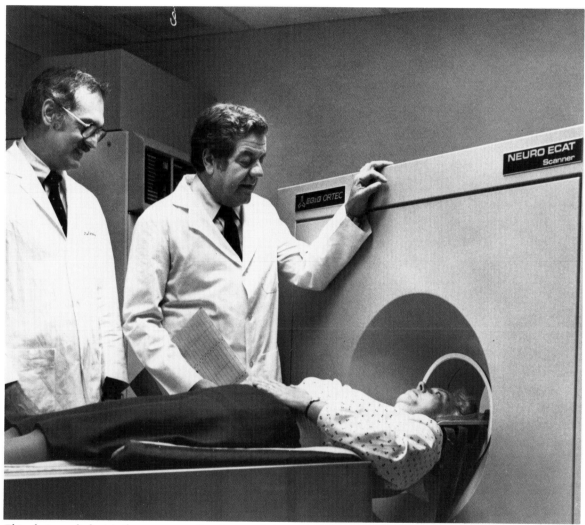

This photograph depicts the recent use of positron emission tomography in medicine.

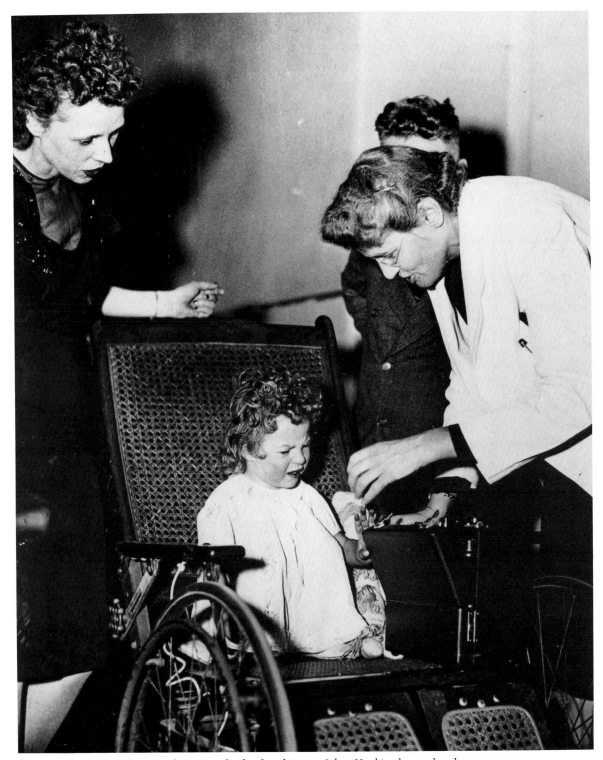

Despite technological advances, the personal side of medicine at Johns Hopkins has endured. The photograph shows Helen B. Taussig with one of her patients, a "blue baby," ca. 1945. Note the child's cyanotic lips and fingertips. The black box Taussig is carrying is a hearing aid; she was partially deaf at the time.

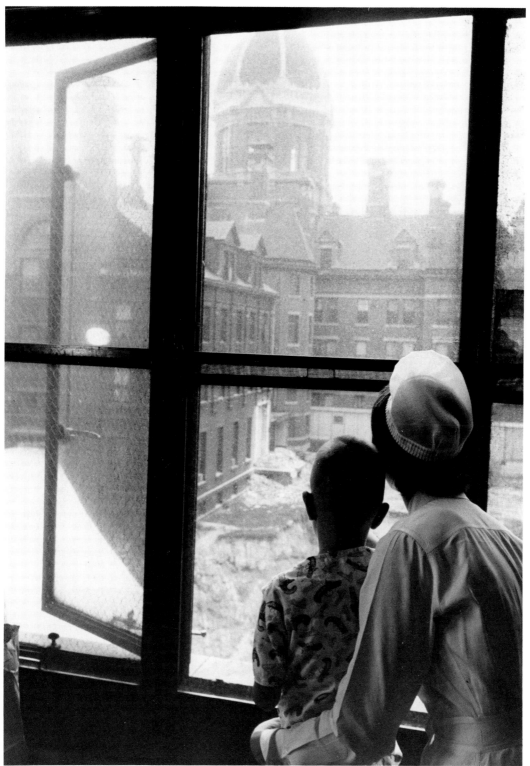

In this photograph, taken in 1962, a pediatric nurse and a young patient hospitalized for cardiac surgery watch the construction of the new Children's Medical and Surgical Center from the third-floor porch of the Halsted Building.

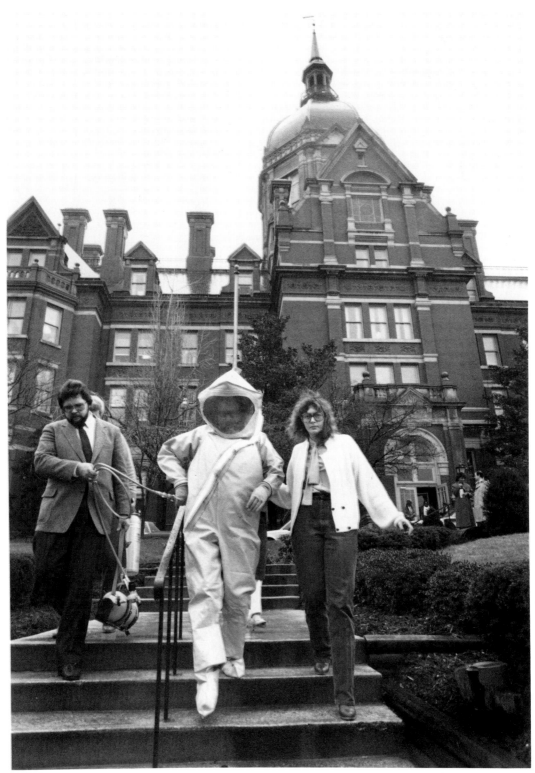

Almost a century after the opening of the hospital, a patient with a rare blood disorder, who was vulnerable to the mildest temperature changes, leaves the hospital in a suit provided by NASA, the National Aeronautics and Space Administration.

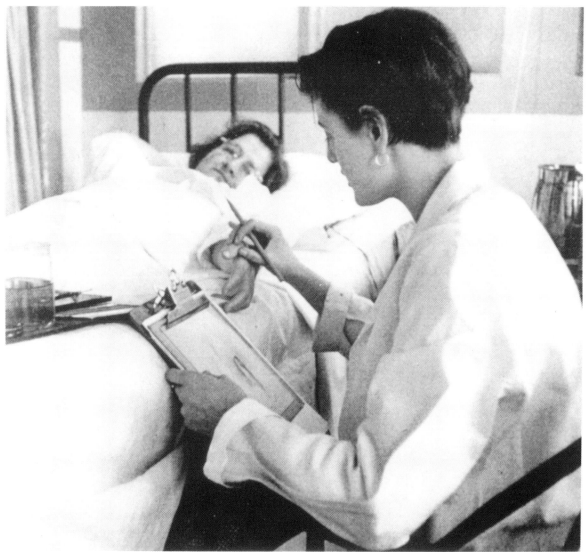

Patients and students meet at the bedside in many different contexts. Here, a student in the program in Art as Applied to Medicine in 1953 works from life. The program was founded in 1921 with Max Broedel at its head.

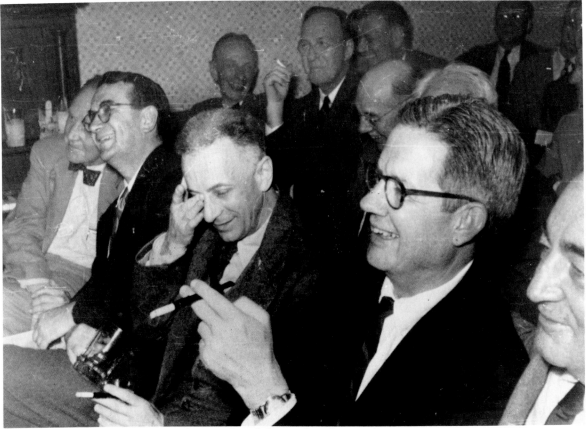

Faculty members in the 1950s at a Pithotomy Show: left to right, Alan M. Chesney, A. McGehee Harvey, Arnold R. Rich, and Alfred Blalock.

Two weeks later, on June 15th, came the commencement exercises of the first graduating class from the medical school, fifteen in all, the majority of whom were to remain another year as house officers or as assistants in one or another of the laboratories. A group of these students had organized what was known as "the Pithotomy Club," a term which indicates the making of a hole in a keg, and there had been festive occasions with song and refreshments in which students and teachers had participated, and in which the foibles of the teachers in particular were not spared in burlesque. Those were indeed informal days at the Hopkins.

—Harvey Cushing[1]

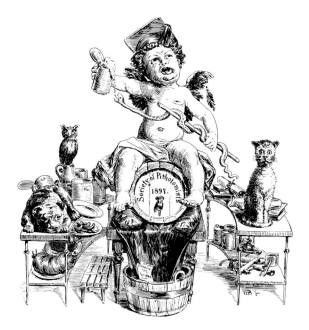

Max Broedel's drawing for the Pithotomy Club.

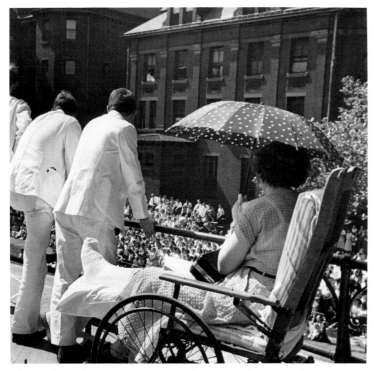

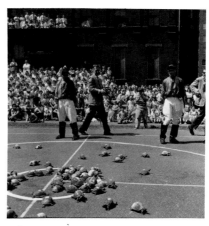

*The Turtle Derby, 1953. Since 1931, thousands of terrapins have competed in this contest,
which has become an elaborate annual hospital event. It has traditionally been held on
the tennis court, first behind the Administration Building, and since the late 1950s, behind
Reed Hall.*

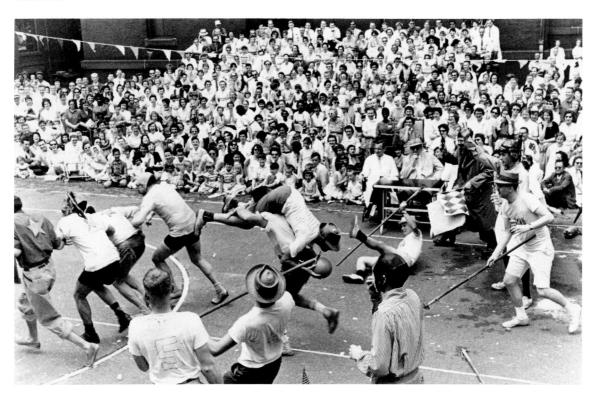

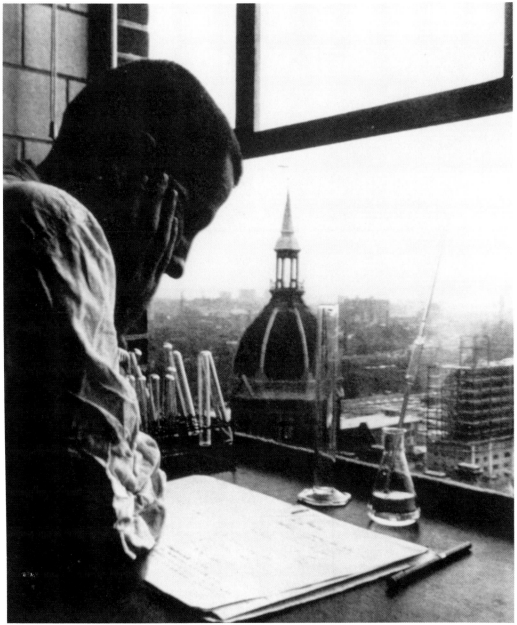

A student contemplates his research notes in 1962. This particular student, John Cameron, became the hospital's surgeon-in-chief.

Given the sacred hunger and proper preliminary training, the student-practitioner requires at least three things with which to stimulate and maintain his education, a notebook, a library, and a quinquennial brain-dusting. I wish I had time to speak of the value of notetaking. You can do nothing as a student in practice without it. Carry a small notebook which will fit into your waistcoat pocket, and never ask a new patient a question without notebook and pencil in hand.

—William Osler[2]

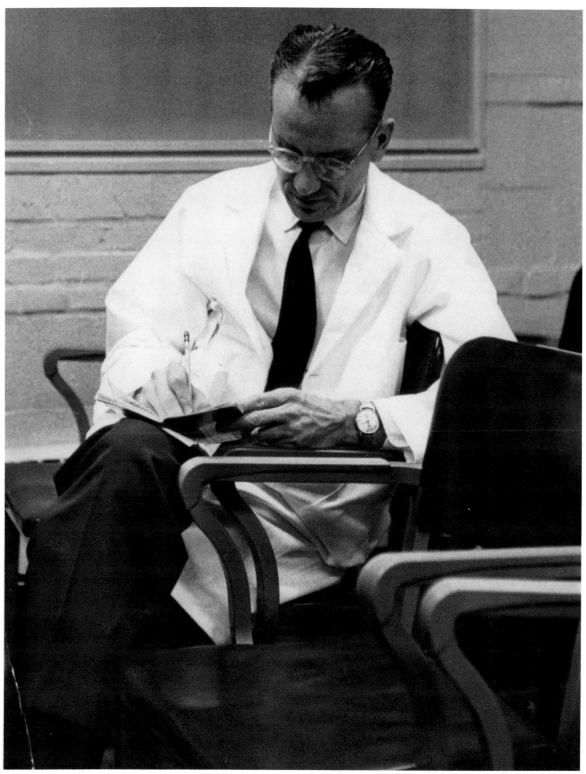

Notetaking is a life-long habit. This photograph shows Hopkins heredity at work. An inveterate notetaker, Victor A. McKusick is never without his notebook handy.

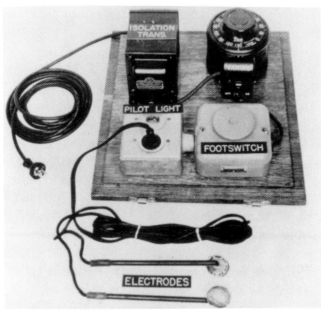

In research, advances in technology included the development of defibrillating equipment and the working out of cardiopulmonary resuscitation techniques. Open (top) and closed (bottom) chest defibrillators were developed by William Kouwenhoven and his colleagues from medicine and surgery.

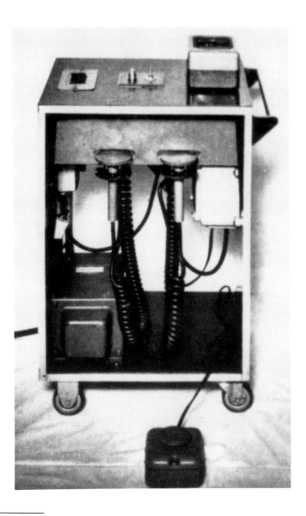

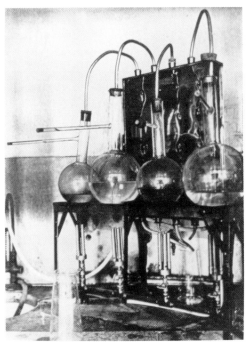
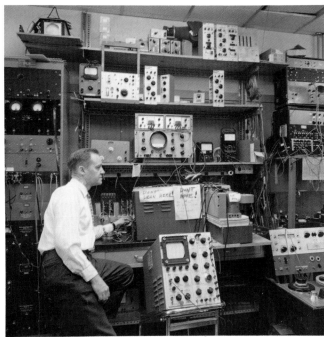

The old science and the new. Above left, chemistry ca. 1915. Large distilling flasks and block tin condensing tubes deliver triply distilled water into the same Jena glass beaker. Above right, George Webb in the Division of Biomedical Engineering's electronics shop, in 1964. Below, P. Shenbaramurthi, a member of the Department of Biological Chemistry, in the Protein/ Peptide Analysis Laboratory opened in 1986.

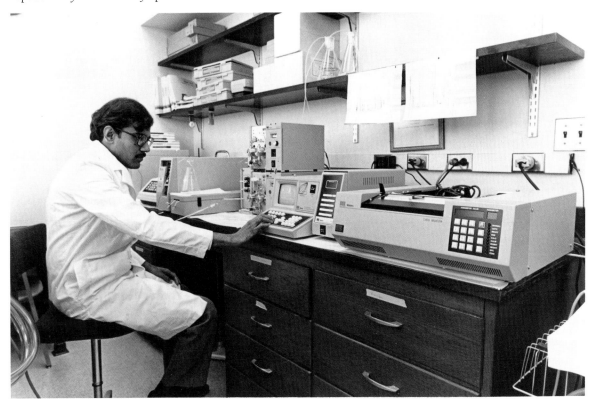

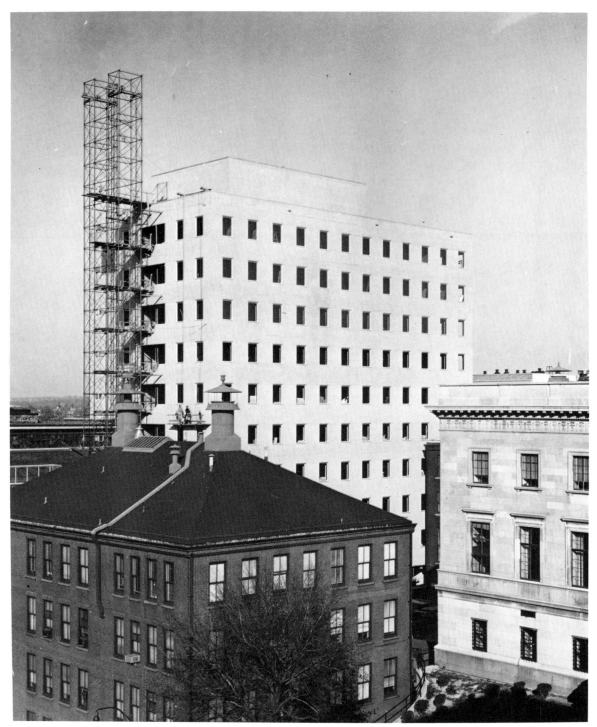

The building boom in the years after World War II utterly changed the face of the East Baltimore campus. New technology required new spaces to enclose it. In the foreground is the Women's Fund Memorial Building, and to the right is the Welch Library. The photograph above shows the Wood Basic Science Building under construction. The photographs on the facing page document the construction of the Biophysics Building on Washington Street, in 1960.

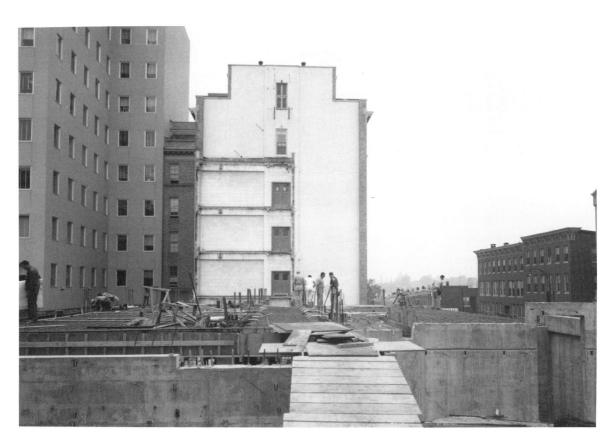

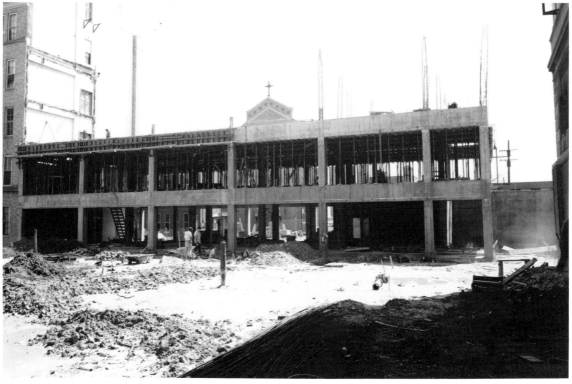

Housing for students and residents was built on McElderry Street and Broadway across from the main entrance to the hospital in 1957.

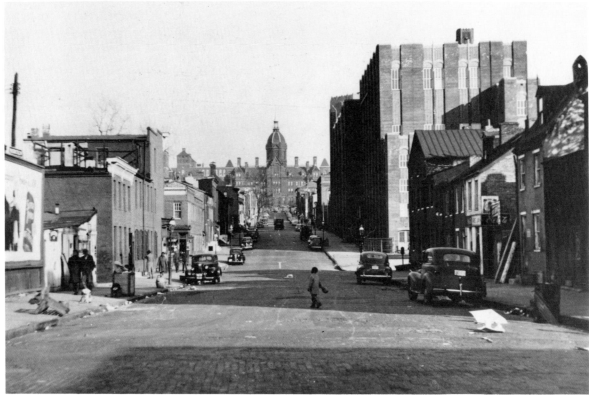

McElderry Street before the construction of this housing.

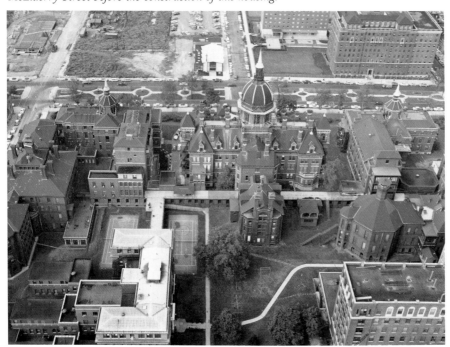

Preparation for construction of 550 North Broadway, upper left.

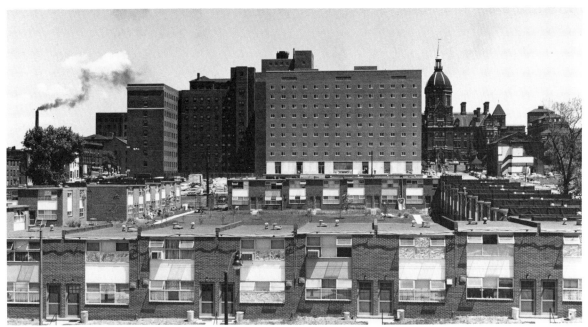

*This photograph, taken in 1957, shows the Broadway Apartments, known as the "Compound,"
in the foreground, and the thirteen-story Reed Hall beyond.*

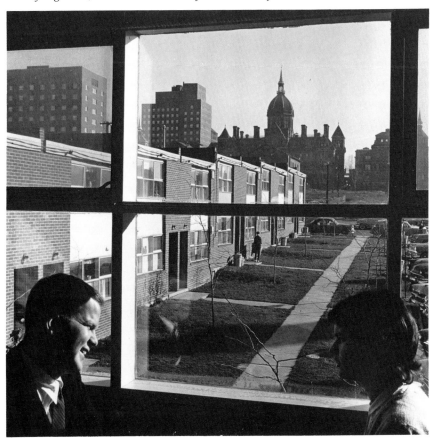

A view of the hospital from within the Compound in 1959.

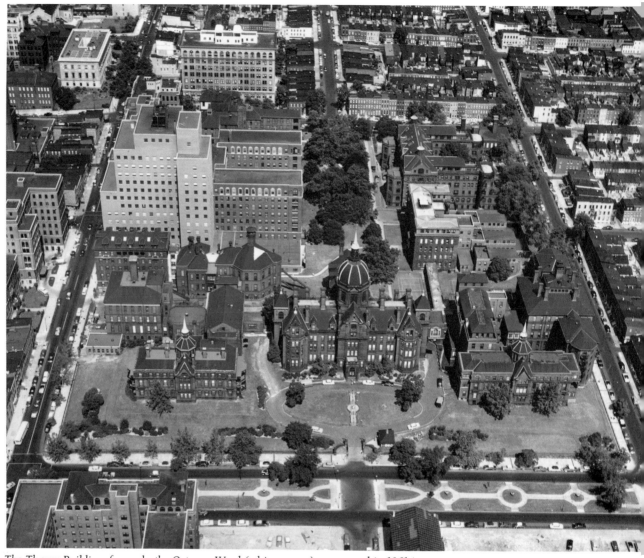

The Thayer Building, formerly the Octagon Ward (white arrow), was razed in 1961 in preparation for construction of the Children's Medical and Surgical Center.

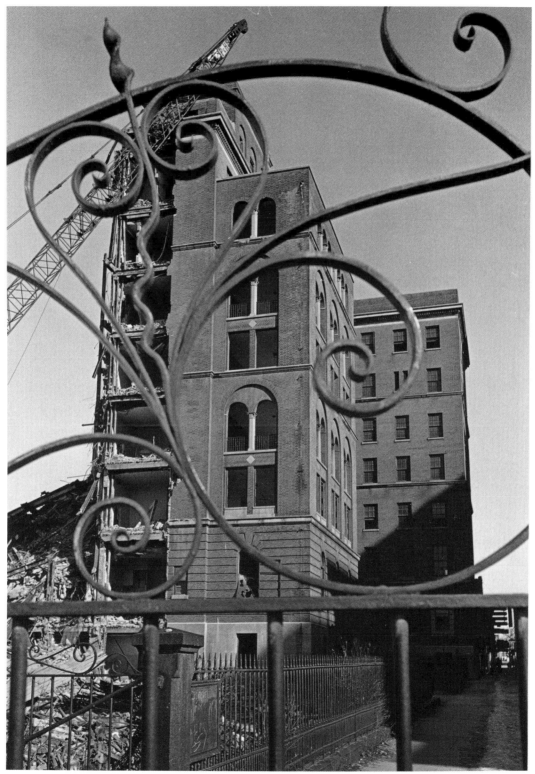

This photograph shows the demolition of the old Sinai Hospital, at Monument Street and Broadway, when Sinai Hospital moved to a more spacious site in the north of Baltimore City.

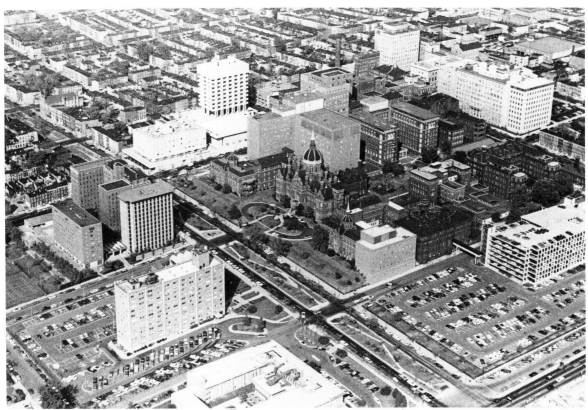

The Kennedy Institute for Handicapped Children and the Turner Auditorium complex, shown here ca. 1968 (white buildings, left upper quadrant), occupy the Sinai lot.

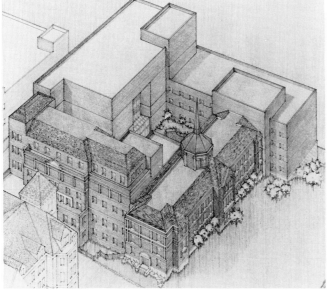

Despite extensive renovation and new construction, parts of the original hospital buildings designed by John Shaw Billings can still be identified, as shown by this 1985 illustration of the Wilmer Institute. Its cluster of buildings form a complete circle that includes the original Female Pay Ward in the foreground (see p. 130).

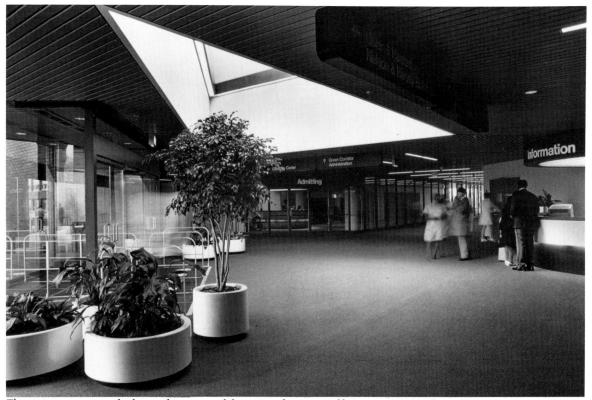

The main entrance to the hospital was moved from Broadway to Wolfe Street in 1979. The triangular skylight is a modern echo of the vaulted ceiling under the dome that had marked the entrance for visitors.

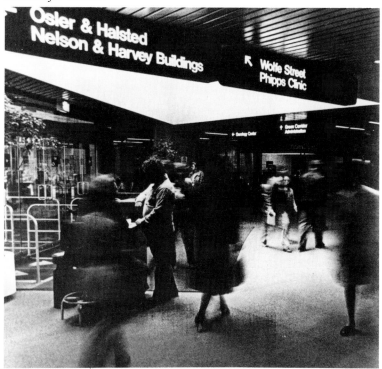

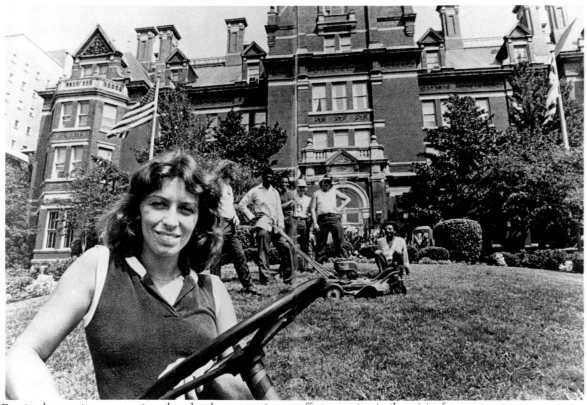

Despite the massive construction, there has been a continuous effort to maintain the spirit of the founder's wishes (see section 1). Trees planted to fill the bare ground in front of the hospital have grown as high as the roof. A grounds crew maintains the plants, grass, and trees around the hospital and in its interior courtyards.

I wish the large grounds surrounding the Hospital Buildings to be properly enclosed by iron railings and to be so laid out and planted with trees and flowers as to afford solace to the sick and be an ornament to the section of the city in which the grounds are located.

—Johns Hopkins[3]

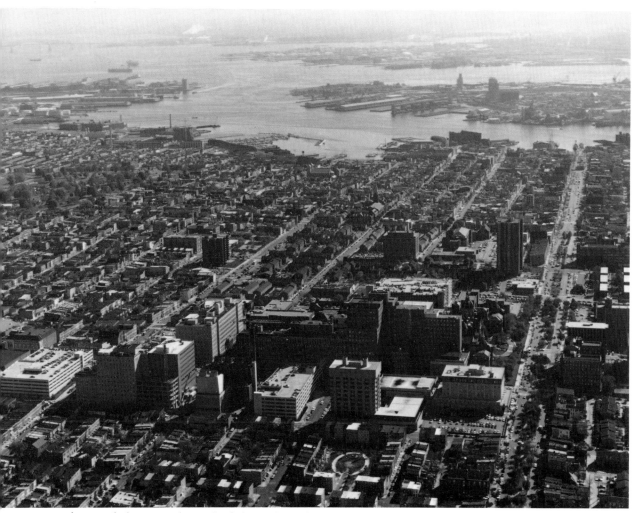

Looking south down Broadway (divided street on right) to the Baltimore Harbor. The original entrance to the hospital (to the right of the photograph) is an isolated oasis of green. The Traylor Building and Turner Auditorium complex appear center foreground. The Hunterian III, completed in 1988, is halfway built (left, foreground).

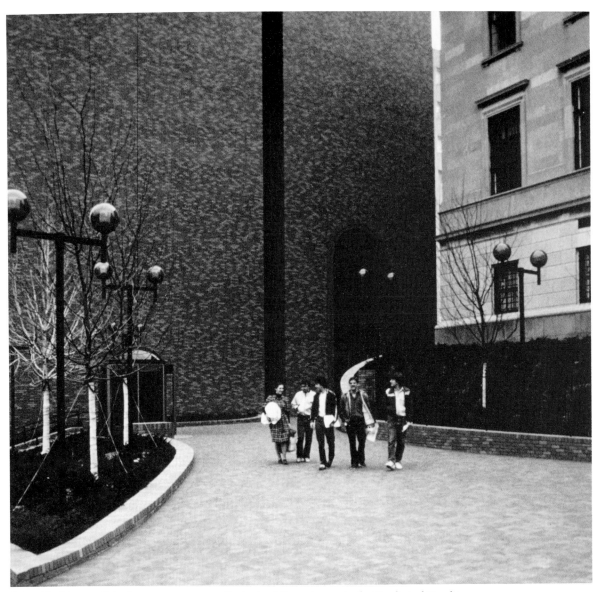

Johns Hopkins medicine's greatest resource: Students at the entrance to the Preclinical Teaching Building.

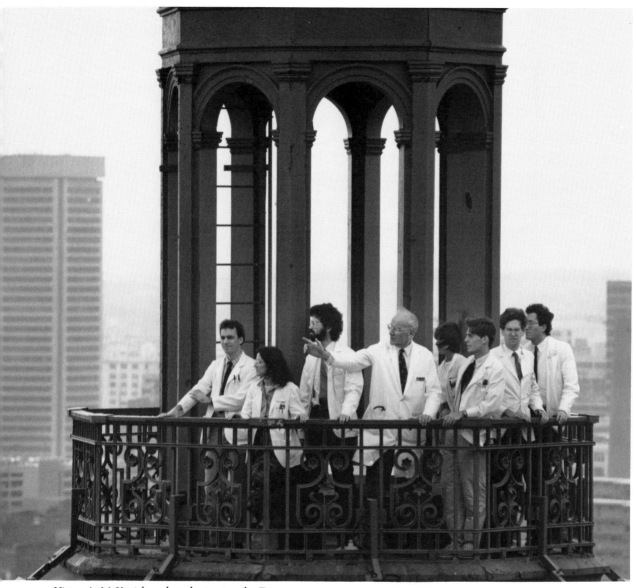

Victor A. McKusick and students atop the Dome.

NOTES

Introduction

1. Quoted in Susan Sontag, *On Photography* (New York: Dell, 1977), p. 185.

2. James Agee, *Let Us Now Praise Famous Men* (Boston: Houghton Mifflin, 1939), p. 13.

3. Alan Gregg, "Dr. Welch's Influence on Medical Education," *Bull. Johns Hopkins Hosp.* 87, suppl. (1950): 28.

4. John Collier, Jr., and Malcolm Collier, *Visual Anthropology: Photography as a Research Method* (Albuquerque: University of New Mexico Press, 1986), p. 45.

5. John D. Stoeckle and George A. White, *Plain Pictures of Plain Doctoring* (Cambridge: MIT Press, 1985); Pete Daniel, Merry A. Foresta, Mamert Stange, and Sally Stein, *Official Images: New Deal Photography* (Washington, D.C.: Smithsonian Institution, 1987).

6. Neil Harris, "Iconography and Intellectual History: The Half-Tone Effect," in *New Directions in American Intellectual History,* ed. John Higham and Paul K. Conkin (Baltimore: Johns Hopkins University Press, 1979), pp. 196–211.

7. Reese V. Jenkins, *Images and Enterprise: Technology and the American Photographic Industry, 1839–1925* (Baltimore: Johns Hopkins University Press, 1975).

8. John A. Kouwenhoven, "Photographs as Historical Documents," in *Half a Truth Is Better than None* (Chicago: University of Chicago Press, 1982), p. 192; Daniel M. Fox and Christopher Lawrence, *Photographing Medicine* (New York: Greenwood Press, 1988).

1. The Opening of the Johns Hopkins Hospital, 1889

1. Kenneth Finkel, *Nineteenth Century Photography in Philadelphia* (New York: Dover, 1980).

2. From a review in the *Nation*, Feb. 5, 1891, quoted by F. H. Szasz and R. F. Bogardus, "The Camera and the American Social Conscience: The Documentary Photography of Jacob A. Riis," *New York Hist.* 55 (1974): 428.

3. Henry M. Hurd, "A History of the First Quarter Century of the Johns Hopkins Hospital," unpublished ms.

4. Gert H. Brieger, "The Original Plans for the Johns Hopkins Hospital and Their Historical Significance." *Bull. Hist. Med.* 39 (1965): 518–28.

5. Caspar Morris, in *Five Essays Relating to the Construction, Organization, and Management of Hospitals* (New York: William Wood, 1875), p. 183.

6. Hurd, "A History of the First Quarter Century."

7. John S. Billings, *Description of the Johns Hopkins Hospital* (Baltimore: Johns Hopkins Hospital, 1890), pp. 36–37.

8. William Osler, "The Natural Method of Teaching the Subject of Medicine," *JAMA* 36 (1901): 1673–79.

9. William Osler, "Specialism in the General Hospital," *Johns Hopkins Hosp. Bull.* 24 (1913): 169.

10. Rufus Cole, "Sir William Osler, Teacher and Student," *Bull. IX of the Internat. Assoc. Med. Museums* (1926), pp. 46–51; p. 49.

11. Edith Gittings Reid, *The Life and Convictions of William Sydney Thayer* (London: Oxford University Press, 1936), p. 55.

12. Thomas B. Turner, *Part of Medicine, Part of Me* (Baltimore: Johns Hopkins University School of Medicine, 1981), p. 141.

13. Hunter Robb, quoted in Harvey Cushing, *The Life of Sir William Osler,* 2 vols. (London: Oxford University Press, 1940), 1:349.

14. William T. Councilman, second member appointed to the faculty in pathology, later professor of pathology at Harvard, quoted in Cushing, *Life of Osler,* 1:317.

15. Daniel C. Gilman, 1896, cited by Nancy McCall, "The Statue of the Christus Consolator at the Johns Hopkins Hospital: Its Acquisition and Historic Origins," *Johns Hopkins Med. J.* 151 (1982): 13.

16. John S. Billings, *The Johns Hopkins Hospital: Reports and Papers Relating to Construction and Organization*, no. 1 (1876): 15.

17. Billings, "Description of the Johns Hopkins Hospital," p. 39.

18. Recounted in Ethel Johns's preparatory notes for a later published history of the nursing school at Johns Hopkins, The Johns Hopkins Nurses' Alumnae Office, Robb Hall, Baltimore, MD, p. 90. Cited in Nancy Louise Noel, "Isabel Hampton Robb: Architect of American Nursing." Dissertation, D.Ed., Teacher's College, Columbia University, 1979.

2. The Early Years of the Johns Hopkins University School of Medicine, 1893–1914

1. Johns Hopkins, letter to trustees, 1873, in Alan M. Chesney, *The Johns Hopkins Hospital and The Johns Hopkins University School of Medicine*, 3 vols. (Baltimore: Johns Hopkins Press, 1943–63), 1:16.

2. William H. Welch, "The Johns Hopkins Medical School," in Announcement of the Johns Hopkins Medical School (Baltimore: The Johns Hopkins Press, 1893).

3. John Shaw Billings, "Description of The Johns Hopkins Hospital" (Baltimore: Johns Hopkins Hospital, 1890), p. 45.

4. Franklin P. Mall, "The Anatomical Course and Laboratory of the Johns Hopkins University," *Johns Hopkins Hosp. Bull.* 7 (1896): 85.

5. A. S. Murray, "Photography Applied to Surgery," *Johns Hopkins Hospital Reports* 3 (1894): 123.

6. E. M. K. Geiling, "John Jacob Abel, Decade, 1923–1932," *Bull. Johns Hopkins Hosp.* 101, no. 6 (1957): 317. Geiling is quoting from a letter written by one of Abel's associates who joined the department in 1926. The letter writer is not identified.

7. Harvey Cushing, "Instruction in Operative Medicine," *Johns Hopkins Hosp. Bull.* 17 (1906): 123–34, pp. 128.

8. Ibid., pp. 127, 128, 132.

9. Ibid., pp. 124, 126.

10. Royal Cortissoz, The Johns Hopkins University Circular, February 1907. Quoted in "The Four Doctors," *Johns Hopkins Alumni Magazine* (1913–14), 2:23–26.

3. The Hospital's First Twenty-five Years, 1889–1914

1. Alan M. Chesney, *The Johns Hopkins Hospital and the Johns Hopkins University School of Medicine*. 3 vols. (Baltimore: Johns Hopkins Press, 1943–63), 3:280.

2. "Remarks of Judge Harlan," *Johns Hopkins Hosp. Bull.* 25 (1914): 352–53.

3. William Osler, "Looking Back," *Johns Hopkins Hosp. Bull.* 25 (1914): 354–55.

4. Howard A. Kelly, "The Gynecological Operating Room in the Johns Hopkins Hospital, and the Antiseptic and Aseptic Rules in Force," *The Johns Hopkins Hospital Reports* 2 (1891): 131.

5. Ibid., p. 133.

6. Letter, William Osler to President Ira Remsen, September 1, 1911. Alan Mason Chesney Medical Archives, The Johns Hopkins Medical Institutions.

7. William Osler, "The Natural Method of Teaching the Subject of Medicine," *JAMA* 36 (1901): 1673–79, p. 1675.

8. "Opening of the Surgical Building and New Clinical Amphitheatre of the Johns Hopkins Hospital," *Johns Hopkins Hosp. Bull.* 15 (1904): 379–86.

9. Letter, J. M. T. Finney to G. M. Smith, December 1, 1937, in John F. Fulton, *Harvey Cushing* (Springfield, Ill.: Charles C Thomas, 1946), pp. 237–38.

10. Josephine A. Dolan, *Nursing in Society* (Philadelphia: W. B. Saunders Co., 1978), p. 239. See also Philip A. Kalisch and Beatrice J. Kalisch, *The Advance of American Nursing*, 2d ed. (Boston: Little Brown & Co., 1986), pp. 214–16.

11. Samuel J. Crowe, "Personal Recollections of Dr. Halsted," *Surgery* 32, no. 3 (1952): 461.

12. Joseph C. Bloodgood, "Halsted Thirty-Six Years Ago," *Am. J. Surg.* 14 (1931): 89–148.

13. Adolf Meyer, "The Henry Phipps Psychiatric Clinic," *Johns Hopkins Alumni Magazine* 1 (1912–1913): 289–90.

14. Ibid., pp. 290–91.

4. The Building Boom of the 1920s

1. Henry S. Pritchett, quoted in Thomas B. Turner, *Heritage of Excellence* (Baltimore: Johns Hopkins University Press, 1974), p. 138.

2. M. Elliott Randolph and Robert B. Welch, *The Wilmer Ophthalmological Institute, 1925–1975* (Baltimore: Williams & Wilkins, 1976), p. 32.

5. The Years after World War II

1. Harvey Cushing, *The Life of Sir William Osler.* 2 vols. (London: Oxford University Press, 1940), 1:453.

2. William Osler, *The Student Life: A Farewell Address to Canadian and American Medical Students* (Oxford: Horace Hart, Printer to the University, n.d.), p. 20.

3. Johns Hopkins, letter to the university trustees, March 10, 1873.

ILLUSTRATION CREDITS

Pages 8, 9, 13, 16, 18, 19, 22, 23, 24, 30, 31, 34, 35, 36, 37 (*top*), 42 (*bottom*), 43, 47, 48, 49 (*top*), 50, 54, 55 (*top*), 56, 57, 58, 59, 60, 61, 63, 64, 65, 72 (*bottom*), 73, 75 (*bottom*), 77, 78, 79, 80, 81, 82 (*bottom*), 83 (*top and bottom left*), 84 (*top*), 85 (*top left*), 88, 89, 90 (*top*), 91 (*top*), 92, 94, 99, 100, 102 (*top*), 103, 105, 107, 108, 109, 111 (*bottom*), 112, 114, 115 (*top*), 116 (*top*), 117, 119, 121, 127 (*bottom*), 128 (*top*), 133, 134, 135, 140, 142, 146, 147, 152, 153, 154, 155, 156, 157, 158 (*top*), and 159: The Alan M. Chesney Medical Archives, the Johns Hopkins Medical Institutions.

Pages 10, 11, 12, 14, 15, 17, 26, 27, 28, 29, 32, 33, 38, 39, 40, 41, and 42 (*top*): Frederick Gutekunst, in John Shaw Billings, *Description of the Johns Hopkins Hospital* (Baltimore: The Johns Hopkins Hospital, 1890).

Page 20: Courtesy of the Medical and Chirurgical Faculty of Maryland.

Page 21: John F. Fulton, *Harvey Cushing: A Biography* (Springfield, Ill.: Charles C Thomas, 1946), opposite p. 244.

Pages 25 (*top right and bottom*), 93, and 120 (*bottom*): The Allan Erskine album, the Alan M. Chesney Medical Archives, the Johns Hopkins Medical Institutions.

Page 25 (*top left*): The Murray Shulman album, the Alan M. Chesney Medical Archives, the Johns Hopkins Medical Institutions.

Page 37 (*bottom*): Ed Thorsett, "Hopkins News," *Johns Hopkins Magazine* 28 (March 1977): 32.

Page 46: The *Johns Hopkins Hospital Bulletin* 1 (1889): 1.

Page 49 (*bottom*): National Library of Medicine, Bayne-Jones Papers.

Pages 51 and 52: Franklin P. Mall, "The Anatomical Course and Laboratory of the Johns Hopkins University," *Johns Hopkins Hospital Bulletin* 7 (1896): opposite pp. 96, 97.

Page 53: A. G. Hoen, "The Photographic Room and Apparatus in the Anatomical Laboratory of the Johns Hopkins Hospital," *Johns Hopkins Hospital Bulletin* 7 (1896): opposite p. 110.

Pages 55 (*bottom*) and 129: Robert M. Mottar, "The Johns Hopkins Idea: A 1951 Portrait," *Johns Hopkins Magazine* 2 (Jan.–Feb. 1951): 42, 24.

Page 62: Harvey Cushing, "Instruction in Operative Medicine," *Johns Hopkins Hospital Bulletin* 17 (1906): opposite p. 132.

Pages 67, 84 (*bottom*), 85 (*top right and bottom*), and 106 (*top*): Dean Lewis, "The Johns Hopkins Hospital, Teaching of Surgery," in *Methods and Problems of Medical Education,* Series 8 (New York: Rockefeller Foundation, 1927), pp. 300, 299, 291, 293.

Page 69: "The Four Doctors, " *Johns Hopkins Alumni Magazine* 2 (1913–14): opposite p. 23.

Pages 72 (*top*), 96 (*bottom*), 97 (*top*), 98, 110, 123 (*top*), and 128: *Within the Gates* (Baltimore: The Alumnae Association of the Johns Hopkins Hospital School of Nursing, 1939).

Pages 74 and 75 (*top*): Frederick Gutekunst (1891), in the Alan M. Chesney Medical Archives, the Johns Hopkins Medical Institutions.

Page 76: William Osler, "The Natural Method of Teaching the Subject of Medicine," *JAMA* 36 (1901): 1676. Copyright 1901, American Medical Association.

Page 82 (*top*): James Mitchell, in the Alan M. Chesney Medical Archives, the Johns Hopkins Medical Institutions.

Page 83 (*bottom right*): Courtesy of W. C. Thomas, Jr.

Pages 86, 87 (*top*), 90 (*bottom*), 118 (*top*), 122, 123 (*bottom*), 124 (*top*), and 125: The Nurses' Alumnae Association album, in the Alan M. Chesney Medical Archives, the Johns Hopkins Medical Institutions.

Page 87 (*bottom*): Courtesy of William Wallace Scott.

Page 91 (*bottom*): *Annual Report of the Johns Hopkins Hospital* (1977): 37.

Page 95: Lawrence Emge, in the Alan M. Chesney Medical Archives, the Johns Hopkins Medical Institutions.

Page 96 (*top*): *Johns Hopkins Alumni Magazine* 1 (1912–13): 290.

Pages 97 *(bottom)* and 138 *(top)*: A. Aubrey Bodine estate, Kathleen Ewing Gallery.

Page 102 *(bottom)*: William G. MacCallum, "The Pathological Laboratory of the Johns Hopkins University and Hospital," in *Methods and Problems of Medical Education,* Series 3 (New York: Rockefeller Foundation, 1925), p. 163.

Pages 104 *(top)* and 148: Robert Phillips, in "The Education of a Physician," *Johns Hopkins Magazine* 15 (Dec. 1963–Jan. 1964): 23, 51.

Page 104 *(bottom)*: Courtesy of the Department of Pathology, the Johns Hopkins University School of Medicine.

Page 106 *(bottom)*: *Thirty-Fifth Report of the Director of the Johns Hopkins Hospital* (Baltimore: Johns Hopkins Press, 1924), between pp. 28 and 29.

Page 111 *(top)*: *Twenty-Fourth Report of the Superintendent of the Johns Hopkins Hospital* (Baltimore: Johns Hopkins Press, 1913), opposite p. 33.

Page 113: *The Johns Hopkins Hospital* (film commemorating the fiftieth anniversary of the opening of the hospital, 1939), courtesy of the Motion Picture and Television Department, the Johns Hopkins University School of Medicine.

Pages 115 *(bottom)* and 116 *(bottom)*: Warfield T. Longcope, "Medical Clinic, Johns Hopkins Hospital," in *Methods and Problems of Medical Education,* Series 11–12 (New York: Rockefeller Foundation, 1928), pp. 67, 73.

Page 120: Alan J. Bearden, "The Pathologist," *Johns Hopkins Magazine* 10 (Nov. 1958): 12.

Pages 124 *(bottom)* and 138 *(bottom)*: Courtesy of Richard S. Ross.

Page 127 *(top)*: Robert M. Mottar, "Interne's Day," *Johns Hopkins Magazine* 2 (April 1951): 16.

Pages 128 *(bottom)*, 131 *(bottom)*, and 151 *(top right)*: Baltimore City Life Museums/The Peale Museum.

Pages 130, 131 *(top)*, and 132 *(top)*: M. Elliott Randolph and Robert B. Welch, *The Wilmer Ophthalmological Institute,*

1925–1975 (Baltimore: Williams & Wilkins, 1976), pp. 37, 168, 34, 48.

Page 132 *(bottom)*: © Peggy Fox, in "The Wilmer Eye Institute at Hopkins," Office of Public Affairs, the Johns Hopkins Medical Institutions, 1985.

Page 139: Jack Engeman, in "The Use of Isotopes in Medicine," *Johns Hopkins Magazine* 2 (Nov. 1950): 12.

Pages 141 and 162: Courtesy of the Office of Public Affairs, the Johns Hopkins Medical Institutions.

Page 143: Robert Phillips, in the Alan M. Chesney Medical Archives, the Johns Hopkins Medical Institutions.

Page 144: © Kevin Webber.

Page 145: Werner Wolff, Black Star, in "Art in Medicine," *Johns Hopkins Magazine* 5 (Oct. 1953): 12–13.

Page 149: Courtesy of J. Michael Criley.

Page 150 *(top)*: William Kouwenhoven, "The Effects of Electricity on the Human Body," *Johns Hopkins Medical Journal* 115 (1964): 430.

Page 150 *(bottom)*: William B. Kouwenhoven et al., "Closed Chest Defibrillation of the Heart," *Surgery* 42(1) (Sept. 1957): 550.

Page 151 *(top left)*: Sydney R. Miller et al., "A Further Study of the Diagnostic Value of the Colloidal Gold Reaction, Together with a Method for the Preparation of the Reagent," *Johns Hopkins Hospital Bulletin* 26 (1915): opposite p. 396.

Page 151 *(bottom)*: Courtesy of Thomas Stiltz.

Page 158 *(bottom)*: RTKL Associates, Inc., in "The Wilmer Eye Institute at Hopkins," Office of Public Affairs, the Johns Hopkins Medical Institutions, 1985.

Page 159 *(bottom)*: Bill Denison, "Making Rounds," *Johns Hopkins Magazine* 32 (June 1981): 12.

Page 160: Richard Anderson, *Annual Report of the Johns Hopkins Hospital* (1980).

Page 161: Vernon Snyder Aerial Photography.

Page 163: © Bill Denison.

INDEX

_____

Page numbers in italic denote illustrations.